Nigel Keith Maybury was born in 1943 and is a retired general and vascular surgeon of wide experience. He trained at Oxford University and St Thomas's Hospital, London. He was a Wellcome Trust research fellow at the Middlesex Hospital, London and later a lecturer in surgery at the University of Leicester. He was appointed as a consultant surgeon at the Royal Albert Edward Infirmary in Wigan, Greater Manchester. He wrote his thesis for a DM from Oxford, on surgery, for duodenal ulcers—a major disease of the 20th century. His previous book published in 2014 was *The End of the Golden Age of General Surgery*, which describes the training and practice of a surgeon in the second half of the 20th century, before the dramatic changes in the practice of surgery that occurred across Europe at the beginning of the new millennium.

To Sara Elisabeth, my wife, for her love, patience and encouragement during the years of writing this book, for she never knew if I was at home or in a distant time and country.

Nigel Keith Maybury

Surgery: An Unfamiliar History

Austin Macauley Publishers™
London • Cambridge • New York • Sharjah

The medical information in this book is not advice and should not be treated as such. Do not substitute this information for the medical advice of physicians. The information is general and intended to better inform readers of their health care. Always consult your doctor for your individual needs.

A CIP catalogue record for this title is available from the British Library.

ISBN 9781398411494 (Paperback)
ISBN 9781398430334 (Hardback)
ISBN 9781398418677 (ePub e-book)

www.austinmacauley.com

First Published 2022
Austin Macauley Publishers Ltd®
1 Canada Square
Canary Wharf
London
E14 5AA

In a book spanning the whole length of civilisation itself, I am indebted to many who lived long ago as well as my contemporaries and friends who have advised and helped in so many ways.

Looking back to the study and interpretation of pre-historic surgery, Dr Guido Majno, is foremost in his description of the surgery of the Peruvians and ancient Egyptians. Also, this book would not be possible without the descriptions of operations first performed in ancient Greece and Rome, by Hippocrates, Celsus and Galen, and also in India by Sustruta. These were later translated by brilliant scholars who made the treatises of the ancients available to a wider public. A window into the surgery of the Middle Ages was provided in books by contemporary surgeons; Ambroise Paré, Thomas Cope, Richard Wiseman and John Hunter. They described the operations of the ancients that they practised during these difficult times. Other valuable sources of information included Dr Donald Campbell's *Arabian Medicine* published in 1926 and a *History of Surgery* by Professor Harold Ellis and many others who are listed in the bibliography.

My grateful thanks go to, Dick Stroud, an author of many books for his erudition and advice; to, Brian Livingstone FRCS, for his attention to surgical detail; to, Neville Lewis, a scholar with a great love of Greece and, Dr David Boase FRCS FRCOpth, for his advice.

Any errors are my responsibility alone.

Foreword

Mr John Black, MD. FRCS. FRCP.
President of the Royal College of Surgeons of England, 2008–2011.

It is difficult to pick up a newspaper without reading about the latest "breakthrough" or even "revolution" in the practice of medicine. However, there is nothing new under the sun and this erudite book illustrates it comprehensively. Starting in 10,000 BC the author not only describes each important advance but sets it into the historical, academic and political context which made it possible, or sometimes impossible. Five ages of surgical progress are defined and it is fascinating to see how surgical ingenuity and the courage to innovate are not confined to our post-enlightenment times. Pioneering surgeons were often ignored or obstructed, but sometimes new techniques spread rapidly, this depending as much on the historical background as on the significance of the advance. External factors such as the religious obstructionism arising from the Papal Edict of Tours of 1163 to the political interference of the European Working Time Directive of early this century are salutary examples.

The author, Keith Maybury, is well suited to his task, having practised as a widely trained and experienced surgeon during the heyday of the British District General Hospital, and having widespread historical and philosophical interests. Because of the wealth of fact and detail this is not a book that will be devoured in one sitting, but it's different approach will fascinate and stimulate not only surgeons but all those interested in medical history.

Table of Contents

Quotation.

The revolution in surgery due to anaesthesia, asepsis, radiography and other practical and scientific progress tends to the modern surgeon being rather out of touch with the great ancients.

E.T. Withington. Translator of Hippocrates, Volume III. Loeb Classical Library, Harvard University Press, 1984.

Previous Publication.

The End of the Golden Age of General Surgery, 1870–2000. The Training and Practice of a General Surgeon in the Late Twentieth Century. By Nigel Keith Maybury. CreateSpace, Printed by Amazon. ISBN: 14995531370. ISBN: 13: 9781499531374. Library of Congress Number: 2014908865. 2014.

Chapter 1
A New Perspective of Surgery

No part of Ancient History is older or more fascinating than the history of surgery that began twelve millennia ago. The first operation was trephination of the skull, a surprising and sophisticated start. The last passed virtually unnoticed and was a complex transplant operation that marked the final triumph of operative surgery, for with this operation all the organs and tissues of the body had finally been successfully operated on, excised or in this case transplanted.

The progress of operative surgery has not been a smooth progression. But there are times in the course of history that have favoured their development. If these periods were identified, a clearer understanding of the circumstances that made them possible could be revealed.

Traditional histories of surgery naturally concentrate on improvements in operations that show the progressive nature of surgery. They briefly acknowledge the surgeons of antiquity, but concentrate on the improvements that took place in medieval and modern times, demonstrating the ever-increasing sophistication in operating technique and the consequent benefits to patients. It is this progress in the improvements made in surgery over time that are rightly emphasised.

The author of this book fully accepts this traditional approach to the history of surgery as described above, but has a different objective. The intention here has been to discover the dates, places and surgeons who were the first to perform an entirely new operation, now renamed as an 'original operation'. This was to clearly differentiate them from later improvements and modifications and the need to do this will be explained. Meantime, a search from early antiquity to the present was undertaken to identify 'original operations'. This was successful and the result is Figure 1.1, that identifies the dates and civilisations that were favourable or unfavourable to the undertaking and production of original operations.

Contemporary descriptions of original operations have survived, with less than ninety being identified. Each of these is also a 'generic' procedure and embraces a larger group or class of similar operations that are derived from it over the course of time. As the discovery of original operations has been fundamental to this book, each has been described, fixing it in time and space. Its subsequent history of improvements is also described, confirming the uniqueness of original operations and how they have moulded all of surgery from antiquity to the present. These are presented in chapters for each period.

Also revealed by the timeline is a period of 1,300 years when no original operations were undertaken. This followed the fall of the Western Roman Empire up to the late Middle Ages. This unexpected and lengthy period without any original operations is analysed and reasons for its occurrence and its consequences presented in later chapters.

To achieve this, a timeline recording only original operations needed to be established. This involved the exclusion of subsequent modifications and improvements to develop a clear picture of the times and countries that were favourable for the undertaking of original operations.

An example from the 5th century BC records a description by Hippocrates of how to trephine the skull.[1] It seemed reasonable to assume that this was one of his original operations, as the ancients did not usually quote their sources. However, radiocarbon studies in the 20th century revealed that trephinations of the skull originated in Peru in about 10,000 BC, predating Hippocrates by over 9,000 years. It is now known that its practise slowly spread from there through North America and across Eurasia over several thousand years. The last known trephination by an indigenous surgeon was in Morocco in the late 19th century. Hippocrates[2] must have known of the pre-existence of this operation as he modified and improved it, so making him a 'successor surgeon' to the Peruvian's 'original operation'. It is now recorded as the first original operation in Figure 1.1. Further modifications were made to it by Celsus[3] in the 1st century AD and again by Galen[4] in the 2nd century, so confirming that repeated improvements are common and have continued to this day. It may seem puzzling why such a seemingly complex operation, as trephination of the skull was the first of all the original operations. The author[5] can vouch that trephination of the skull is not a technically difficult operation to perform once properly learned and taught, but still attests to the skill of those early surgeons.

Another example of differentiating an original operation from modifications made by later surgeons is the operation for fistula. A common complaint of men who spent much time in the saddle. The surgical cure was described by John of Arderne[6] in the 14th century, when he was then considered the 'Father of Surgery' in England, for this operation was attributed to him. However, Hippocrates had written a clear description of how to carry out this operation 1800 years earlier and his description is in all respects the same operation as practised today. The original operation for fistula is therefore attributed to Hippocrates and not John of Ardern who had earlier attended Montpellier University where Hippocrates treatises were available for study.

Another generic original operation was the insertion of an arterial bypass graft. This was first carried out in 1948 on a patient at risk of developing gangrene of a leg, due to the occlusion of the femoral artery. This blockage was 'bypassed' by using the patient's own long saphenous vein, harvested from the same leg and used as a substitute artery. This successfully restored the circulation in the leg. Twelve years later in 1960, the first coronary artery bypass graft was also a success. Although it was a new operation, it does not qualify as an original operation, because the cardiac surgeon knew in advance that a successful outcome could be achieved using a technique that had previously been proved successful in a leg.

True novelty in any great endeavour, including surgery, is rare and surgeons who devised and carried out original operations were the trailblazers of surgical practice, they exhibited both the necessary skill and the determination to develop and carry out these operations. Their endeavours were often accompanied by objections and active discouragement from colleagues.

An example of this took place in the 1950s. The surgeon involved had developed and replaced cataracts in the eye by a lightweight thermoplastic implant made of Perspex. Its success has resulted in millions of patients with cataracts having their sight restored. The surgeon was Mr Harold Lloyd Ridley (1906–2001),[8] a specialist in ophthalmology. He had treated wounded Royal Air Force pilots during World War II. One pilot had suffered trauma to an eye, when the Perspex windscreen of his plane had been shattered by enemy cannon fire. Ridley noted that this particular foreign body in the eye was not infected nor had it particularly obscured the pilot's vision. He took note and after the war spent many years pioneering the development of a synthetic lens. He worked against strong opposition and discouragement from the medical communities of both England and the USA. Finally, his work was publicly recognised and he was made a Fellow of the Royal Society of London in 1986 and awarded a knighthood.

This demonstrates that trailblazers have to overcome considerable difficulties and challenges that any truly original work requires. It is only when these high barriers have been successfully surmounted, that later generations of surgeons who copy and update original operations are secure and comforted in the knowledge that these operations have already been successfully carried out. For success, including the survival of the patient, are key criteria to give successor surgeons confidence that updating, modifying and improving an original operation would also be successful and of benefit to patients.

Figure 1.1

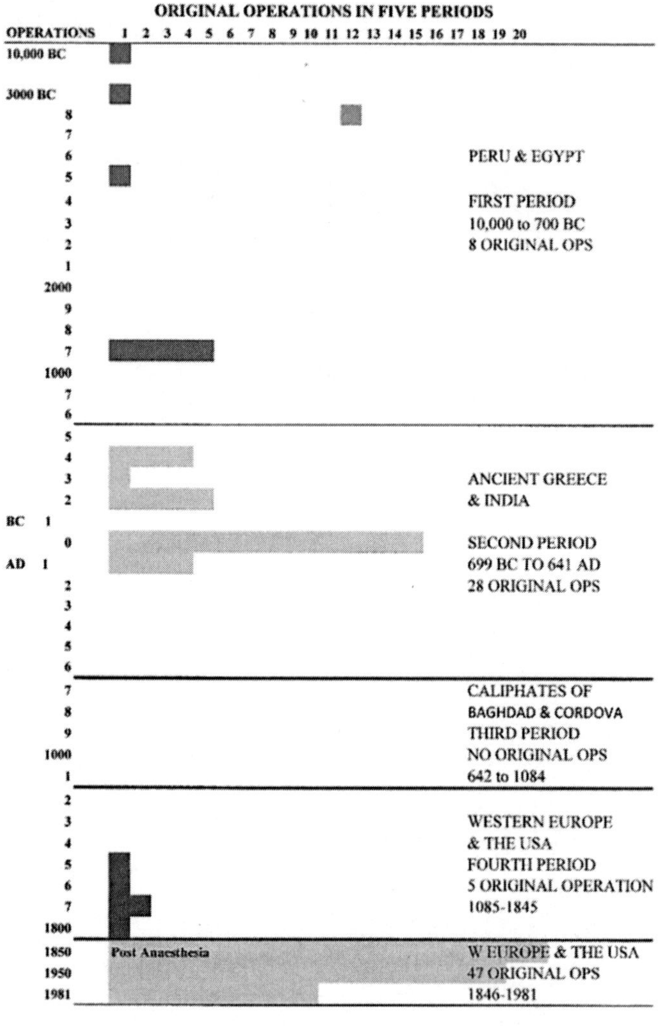

Figure 1.1. *The only way to discover surgeons who undertook original operations was to search the surgical literature. The result was this schematic timeline that divides into five periods beginning in 10,000 BC and ending in 1981. Each period is separated by a dark line. The numbers of operations in each period are represented by the horizontal bars, which are coloured black and grey to differentiate the five periods. A total of 88 original operations have been identified. Eight in the first period, 28 in the second, none in the third, five in the fourth and 47 in the fifth period.*

The result of identifying and placing only original operations in the timeline above was successful in establishing a clear pattern to their distribution. It shows that in four of the five periods demonstrated, two of them, the second and the fifth show surgical genius at its best and encompassed 85% of all original operations. The first and fourth periods only amounted to 15% of the original operations and none were found in the third period. The subsequent detailed analysis of the complex conditions that resulted in success or failure of these periods is described.

The next chapter presents a timeline of all the original operations identified. It also gives the chapters where each original operation is described including the operation's subsequent history, so confirming the continuity of surgery over time. These data are the basis of this history and reveal when, where and by whom each took place, enabling a detailed analysis of each of the five periods of surgery to be undertaken.

Notes and References

References to Chapter 2 give the date of each original operation and where the full description of the original operation is to be found.

1. Chapter 2. c10,000 BC. Trephination of the skull.
2. Hippocrates. On wounds of the head. Volume III. Translated by E.T. Withington. Loeb Classical Library, Harvard College, USA. Reprinted 1984. pp. 1–51
3. Celsus on Medicine. Volume III, Books 7–8. Loeb Classical Library. Harvard College, USA. 1938. p. 497.
4. Galen. Method of Medicine. Vol II. Loeb Classical Library. Edited and Translated by Ian Johnston and G.H.R. Horsley. Harvard University Press, 2011, p. 215–251.
5. The End of the Golden Age of General Surgery. 1870–2000. The Training and Practice of a General Surgeon in the Late Twentieth Century. By N.K. Maybury. ISBN 1499531370, ISBN 2014908865. CreateSpace Independent Publishing Platform, North Charleston, South Carolina. 2014, p 28.
6. Chapter 2, Index and Timeline. c425 BC. Original operation attributed to Hippocrates, with John of Arderne as a successor surgeon.

7. Historical Vignetted in Vascular Surgery. The History of in situ saphenous vein bypass. John E. Connolly. Editor Norman M. Rich. J. Vasc. Surg, 2011; 241-4.
8. Chapter 2. The development of synthetic intraocular lenses by Sir Harold Ridley.

Chapter 2

Original Operations Identified and Divided into Five Periods

1. Introduction.
2. First period, c10,000 BC to c700 BC.
3. Second period, 699 BC to 641 AD.
4. Third period, 642 to 1084.
5. Fourth period, 1085 to 1845.
6. Fifth period, 1846 to 1981.

Searching the literature from antiquity to the present yielded 88 generic original operations. Each is listed in this chapter with the year when it was undertaken and the country of origin and naturally divides into five periods of surgery.

The intention of this chapter is to provide an overview and index of how surgery developed, recording its increasing sophistication over time, while clearly illustrating that this was not a smooth progression, for the undertaking of original operations was significantly influenced by many factors that will be described in the course of the book.

In more practical terms, it gives directions of where to find the full description of each original operation and its subsequent modifications and improvements.

All the original operations are shown in bold type, to distinguish them, from the entries on history, anatomy, physiology, relevant political events, advances in technology and science, that are all presented in *Italics.*

Abbreviations.

AD = Anno Domini = Christian or Common Era.

BC = Dates before the Christian or Common Era.

c = circa, about or approximately.

f = flourish, approximate period of best work.

r = dates that a king reigned.

d = date of death.

The First Period, c10,000 BC to c700 BC.

Eight original operations and procedures from Peru and Ancient Egypt

The original operations or procedures are listed below. The main article related to each is in Chapter 3 where the page number is given. It is only in the Egyptian period that 'original procedures' are listed with the original operations, this is because they represent new surgical-techniques that have been used by surgeons ever since, such as suturing wounds and the setting fractures. The date of this first period ends with the beginning of the Greek era.

c10,000 BC. Peru. Trephination of the skull.

c3,000 BC. Egypt. Catheterisation for retention of urine

c2,500 BC. Egypt. Circumcision

c1,700 BC Babylon. Hammurabi's laws governing surgery

c1,700 BC. Egypt. Edwin Smith Papyrus

Splinting of fractured bones

Reduction of a dislocated jaw

Use of sutures to close wounds

Use of cautery

c1,700 BC. Egypt. Surgical incision of abscesses

c1,550 BC. The use of antiseptics

The Second Period. 699 BC to 641 AD.

With 28 original operations from Ancient Greece, India and Rome.

The full articles describing the original operations from this period are to be found in Chapter 5 under the date and page number given with each entry.

The date of 699 BC marks the approximate beginning of Ancient Greek surgery. While 641 AD marks the end of Greek era when the Museum and

Library in Alexandria in Egypt, the last stronghold of Greek philosophy, science and surgery fell to an Arab army.

c425 BC. Greece.
Surgery for fistula-in-ano
Haemorrhoidectomy
Excision of a dead foetus at term
The operation of venesection.
Excision of bladder stones
c320 BC India. The first Caesarean section

c260 BC. Greece. First human dissections

c260 BC. Greece. Erasistratus of Ceos. The heart recognised as a one-way pump

c250 BC Greek. Ctesibius of Alexandria. Advances in technology. The invention of the syringe and pump

c200 BC India.
Snake bites, first use of tourniquet
Plastic surgery. Earlobe reconstruction
Plastic surgery. First nasal reconstruction
Couching of cataracts
c30 AD. Rome.
Ligation of blood vessels
Amputation of limbs
Excision of tonsils
Umbilical hernia repair
Inguinal hernia repair
Operation for varicocele
Operations for Varicose veins
Excision of impacted urethral stone
Suturing of a perforated colon
Reversal of circumcision
Draining abdominal ascites
Partial thyroidectomy
Mastectomy

Hydrocele

c79 AD. Rome. The first hospitals

c120 AD. Rome. First vaginal hysterectomy

c170 AD. Rome. First aneurysmal operation

c170 AD. Rome. First Tracheostomy

c180 AD. Rome

The suture of tendons and muscles

Anatomical advances

First physiological experiments

Wounds healed without sepsis

410. The fall of Rome and the beginning of the Dark Ages in the West

The Third Period from 642 to 1084.
There were no original operations during the Caliphates of Baghdad and Cordova.

The date of 642 is taken for the start of this period and marks the conquest of Egypt by an Arab army that ended the Greek era. The end date of 1084 was when Toledo, a Muslim city in Spain, fell to a Christian army. Toledo was already an important city where Ancient Greek manuscripts had been translated into Arabic. Almost immediately after the city changed hands, Christian scholars, in their turn were soon translating the Arabic treatises into Latin. Therefore, despite the fact that no original operations took place during this third period, it was otherwise a Golden Age of learning, that included translations of the Ancient Greek manuscripts into Syriac and Arabic. These were critical steps in the transfer of Greek philosophy, medicine and surgery that eventually reached Italy and Western Europe. The main articles are to be found in Chapter 9, on the page numbers given after each entry.

Arabian contribution to surgery,

2nd Century BC. Hippocrates. Translations of his manuscripts

c387 BC. The foundation of Plato's Academy

431 AD. The exile of Nestorius from Byzantium

529. The destruction of the Library in Alexandria in Egypt

622. John the Grammarian and Aaron the Presbyter

632 to 732. The Arab conquests

636. The Academy at Gundê-Shäpūr

c640. Paul of Aegina, the last Byzantine surgeon

762. Baghdad becomes the Capital of the Eastern Caliphate

8th Century. The Nestorians in Baghdad

c850. India, Sushruta's Compendium

9th century. Baghdad, The Caliph al Ma'mūn, Abū Ja'far

*9th century. Hunayn ibn-*Ishāq al Ibadi. *The Isogoge*

9th century. Abu Yusef al-Kindi in Baghdad

c900. Razes, the Golden Age in Baghdad

c1025. Avicenna and the Canon of Medicine based on Galen's manuscripts

c1060. Italy. Constantinus Africanus and the translation of Ancient Greek and Arabic medical texts into Latin

1085. Toledo in Spain. A key centre of translations

12th century. Averroes

and the end of liberal thought in Spain

1204. The Fourth Crusade and the sack of Constantinople

1235. The fall of Cordova

c1246. Ibn al-Nafis. The discovery of the pulmonary circulation

1289. The foundation of the University in Montpellier

The Fourth Period from 1085 to 1845

There were five original operations, four from Western Europe in the medieval and early modern periods and one from the United States of America in the early modern period.

1085 was the year when Toledo fell. 1845 represents the end of the medieval and early modern period and is the year before the introduction of anaesthesia.

The full article on each original operation is in Chapter 10, with its page number.

c1088. Italy. The birth of learning in the West, with new universities

1163. France. The Edict of Tours

1252. France. Establishment of Surgical Guilds

1258. Italy. Pus is not laudable

1300. England. From Guild to Company of Surgeons of London

1440. Germany. Printed Books in Europe and the dissemination of knowledge

1506. Italy. The foundation of pathological anatomy

1543. Anatomy becomes a modern science under Vesalius

1575. France. First transurethral prostatectomy

1585. France. European battlefield surgery surpasses Galen

1609. Italy. The compound microscope developed by Galileo Galilei

1628. England. William Harvey proves the circulation of the blood

c1650. France. Partial excision of the tongue

1665. England. First publication and distribution of medical journals

1673. Netherlands. Identification of bacteria

1740. France. The first skin transplant

1768. England. John Hunter. The development of Teaching Hospitals in London

1785. England. The first parotidectomy

1799. England. Foundation of the Hunterian Museum.

1809. USA. First planned laparotomy, excision of ovarian cyst

1840. Poland. The rise of therapeutic nihilism

The Fifth Period from 1846 to 1981

Forty-seven original operations were undertaken in Western Europe and the United States of America.

Anaesthesia was introduced in 1846 and the last of the original operations was in 1981. The full articles are in Chapter 12, and their page numbers are given below.

1846. USA. Introduction of anaesthesia and the beginning of modern surgery

1846. Austria. Hand washing becomes mandatory before examining a patient

1853. USA. Abdominal Hysterectomy

1856. England. Publication of Gray's Anatomy

1858. France. Microorganisms and germ theory of disease confirmed

1860. Switzerland. Total thyroidectomy

1860. England. Foundation of School for Nurses at St Thomas's Hospital, London

1865. England. Introduction of the antiseptic surgical technique of operating

1867. France. First Splenectomy

1869. Germany. First elective nephrectomy

1871. England. Operative treatment for ileocecal intussusception

1873. Austria. First laryngectomy for cancer

1877. Germany. First esophagectomy

1879. Scotland. First successful excision of an intracranial tumour

1879. Germany. First cystoscope with electric light

1879. Germany. First colectomy

1881. Austria. First gastrectomy

1882. Germany. First cholecystectomy

1883. England. Salpingectomy for an ectopic pregnancy

1883. Scotland. Spine and spinal cord operations other than for trauma

1886. Ireland. Excision of a pharyngeal pouch

1887. USA. First appendicectomy

1889. England. First adrenalectomy

1889. England. First excision of the pituitary

1892. England. First internal fixation of fractures

1892. Germany. First successful suture of a perforated Gastric ulcer

1894. England. First excision of an acoustic
neuroma

1895. Scotland. First pneumonectomy

1895. Germany. The visualisation of internal organs. The discovery of X-rays

1896. France. The discovery of radiation

1896. USA. The first arterial reconstruction

1899. USA. Introduction of surgical gloves

1902. England. Introduction of isotonic intra-venous fluids

1903. France. Surgery for cirrhosis and portal vein hypertension

1904. USA. First radical prostatectomy for prostatic cancer

1906. 1906. USA. First repair of an aneurysm and subsequent developments

1906. Moravia. First successful full-thickness corneal transplant

1907. England. First radical excision of a rectal cancer

1907. France. Curative myotomy for infantile pyloric stenosis

1908. Germany. Invention of diathermy (electro-coagulation

1909. Germany. First pancreatic-duodenectomy

1910. Germany. Introduction of laparoscopy and laparoscopic surgery

1912. Germany. Thymectomy

1915. England. Blood transfusion in World War I

1915. England. Surgical treatment of abdominal wounds in times of war

1915. USA. Intra-cranial surgery for missile injuries

1918. England. Total Cystectomy

1919. USA. Hiatus hernia surgery for gastro-oesophageal reflux

1923. USA. Development of angiography

1923. USA. Mitral valve. First successful open-heart operation

1925. Austria. Parathyroidectomy

1929. England. Discovery of penicillin

1929. Germany. Vascular catheterisation and arterial stenting

1935. USA. The discovery of heparin

1940. USA. The visualisation of internal by ultrasound

1943. USA. Vagotomy for chronic duodenal ulcer disease

1943. USA. Fallot's tetralogy, correction of a congenital cardiac anomaly

1943. USA. The dawn of nuclear medicine

1948. France. First arterial bypass graft

1950. England. Eye surgery, first implant of a synthetic intraocular lens

1950. USA. First kidney transplant was first organ transplant

1953. USA. Bariatric surgery

c1955. England/USA. The surgery of myelomeningocele (MMC)

1958. USA. Introduction of flexible fibre-optic endoscopy. Page 249.

1958. USA. Harrington's rods used to treat idiopathic scoliosis

1961. England. First successful total hip replacement

1969. England. Reconstructive gut surgery

1. **Anal sphincter reconstruction**
2. **Use of small bowel pouches to replace an excised rectum, stomach or bladder**

1981. USA. First in-utero foetal surgery

Addendum.

1963. Heart transplant

1963. Liver transplant

1966. Pancreatic transplant

1983. Lung transplant

1984. Computerised tomography

1984. Chemo-radiation for anal cancer

1987. Combined transplant of liver, heart and lung

1987. Magnetic resonance imaging

1993. Thymus

2000. EU Working time directive

2000. Robot assisted operations

1998. Hand transplants

2005. Face transplant

2012. Bilateral arm transplants

2014. Uterine transplant followed by pregnancy

2018. Penile transplant

Chapter 3: First Period

10,000 BC to 700 BC.

Peru and Ancient Egypt

Original Operations in Peru and Ancient Egypt with Their Subsequent Development c10,000 BC Peru. Trephination of the skull.

The 'first' identified original operation was trephination of the skull in Peru. It involved the removal of a small square of the skull by gradually cutting through the bone using a flint or obsidian blade.[1] During the 20th century, over 1,500 trephined skulls, mainly of men, dating from Neolithic times have been discovered in Peru, North America and across Eurasia including China and Russia. In France, 20 were found from about 6,000 BC, then one in Azerbaijan from 400 BC and the last recorded trephine was by an indigenous surgeon in Morocco in the early 1900s.[2]

Most of the 127 Peruvian skulls had been trephined on the left side of the skull and were usually associated with a fracture, thought to have been be caused by a blow to the head, inflicted by a right-handed enemy wielding a club or stone.

Signs of post-operative infection around the trephines were rare as shown by the smooth healing of the bone, indicating a low rate of sepsis in Neolithic times. Many of the men had more than one trephine with an associated healed fracture and must have survived to fight another day.

Over 9000 years later, Hippocrates (460–370 BC), gives the first written description of the diagnosis and treatment for fractures of the skull including trephination.[3]

Aulus Celsus (c25 BC–c50 AD), a Roman encyclopaedist, also described trephination in great detail. The instruments to trephine the skull had been modified and improved with the development of a metal disc with downturned and serrated teeth with a central pin. This was rotated by a bow and cord. Once the serrated edges of the tube had started to cut into the skull, the pin was removed. The trephination continued slowly until a disc of the skull was cut out. Great care was taken to avoid piercing the underlying dura that protects the brain. To do so would frequently lead to infection of the brain, followed by death. He also had made fine sheets of bronze to protect the dura if a wider exposure of the dura was required.[4]

When the Ancient Greek manuscripts reached Western Europe, the extraordinarily successful results achieved in ancient Peru could not be emulated. In the first half of the 19th century, trephination was almost always associated with infection, followed by the death of the majority of patients. The results were so bad that it was abandoned in Europe until after the antiseptic technique of surgery, devised by Joseph Lister, was introduced in 1865.[5]

These stark differences in outcome between Peru, where the population was small and rural and operations infrequent, gave little opportunity for the practitioners to transfer pathogenic bacteria from one person being operated on to the next. This contrasts with the crowded and dirty towns and cities of Europe, where the surgeons wore the same pus be-splattered aprons that guaranteed the spread of sepsis and death in the times before the infection theory of disease was discovered.[6]

There is no evidence in the Edwin Smith Papyrus of about 1,700 BC that the Ancient Egyptians trephined the skull[7]. Speculation why this original operation had been common in Peru is discussed in Chapter 4.

References:

1. *The Healing Hand. Man and Wound in the Ancient World.* By Guido Majno. Harvard University Press 1985.
2. Restak, Richard 2000. Fixing the brain. Mysteries of the mind. Washington DC national Geographic Society. ISBN: 0-7922-7941-7.
3. *Hippocrates. Loeb Classical Library. Volume 111.* Translation by E.T. Withington. Harvard University Press, Reprinted 1984. pp. 7–58.
4. *Celsus on Medicine. Loeb Classical Library. Book VIII.* With an English translation by W.G. Spencer. Harvard University Press. Pages 498–509.
5. Chapter 2. (Lord) Joseph Lister. 1865.
6. *A History of Surgery*. By Harold Ellis. Greenwich
7. Medical Media Ltd. 2001. ISBN 1 84110 023 4. Edwin Smith Surgical Papyrus by James Henry

8. Breasted. Published in Facsimile with translation and Commentary. University of Chicago Press, 1980.

c3,000 BC Ancient Egypt. Catheterisation for retention of urine.

Catheterisation was first recorded in Ancient Egypt, where straw or other tubes of vegetable origin were first used to relieve retention of urine.[1] Celsus (c25 BC–c50 AD) used bronze tubes as catheters and described three of different lengths for men, the longest being fifteen fingers breadth in length and also two catheters of different sizes for women.[2] When repeated and regular catheterisation was necessary, chronic infection of the urinary tract was inevitable, leading to renal failure and death. This was still the mode of treatment well into the 20th century for men suffering from retention due to benign prostatic enlargement. In the days when men wore top hats, a silver catheter could be conveniently carried about in it for use when needed.

References:

1. A Brief History of Urinary Catheters. Urotoday.com
2. *Celsus on Medicine. Loeb Classical Library. Book VIII.* With an English translation by W.G. Spencer. Harvard University Press. Book V Page LX1.

c2,500 BC. Ancient Egypt. Circumcision.

In a tomb drawing of a high-ranking royal-official in Sakkara in ancient Egypt, dated to the twenty-fifth century BC, there is an illustration of two young men undergoing circumcision. This was probably the first elective or planned operation, whether it was for religious or medical reasons is unknown. It appears that the operators used knives fashioned from stone.[1] Herodotus (c490–c425 BC), the great Greek historian of Antiquity had travelled to Egypt and describes the Egyptian practise of circumcision and wrote that: 'Those from other nations who do so, have learned from the Egyptians'.[2]

References:

1. *Science and Secrets of Early Medicine.* By Jurgen Thorwald, translated from the German by Richard and Clara Winston. Published by Thames and Hudson, 1962. P. 53.
2. *Herodotus the Histories.* Penguin Classics. Translated by Alan de Sélincourt. 1954, 358910864. P. 99.

c1,700 BC surgery. Hammurabi (c1,810–1,750 BC), King of Babylon ordered a code of laws to be carved in stone. This stone is now to be found in the Louvre in Paris. On it is prescribed a high reward for medical or surgical success. However, failure could result in the surgeon's hands being cut off, if he had treated a man's wound with a bronze knife and the patient had died.[1]

References:

1. Wikipedia. Code of Hammurabi.

c1,700 BC Ancient Egypt. The Edwin Smith papyrus.

This ancient Papyrus was discovered in Egypt in the 1860s. It documents 48 cases of generic trauma starting with injuries to the head and then in descending order down the body. Information of injuries below the chest has been lost. The only surgical conditions treated were wounds, fractures and dislocations. It is possible that this papyrus is older than originally thought.

The Ancient Egyptian surgeon describes the care he took before treating a patient and he was the first to make a diagnosis in order to calculate the chances of a successful outcome from possible treatment. He did this by classifying the patient's injuries in three categories. 'An ailment that I will treat', 'An ailment with which I will contend' and significantly, 'An ailment not to be treated'. This showed he would not operate or treat a patient who he thought was incurable and who would probably die from his wounds.[1&2]

Reference:

1. *Cambridge Illustrated History of Medicine.* Edited by Roy Porter. Cambridge University Press, 1996. ISBN 0 521 44211. Page 204.

2. *The Healing Hand. Man, and Wound in the Ancient World.* By Guido Majno. Harvard University Press 1985. P. 91.

Splinting of fractured bones. (Edwin Smith Papyrus)

The first splinting of a fractured bone was described as follows. 'The patient is laid on his back in a position to spread apart the upper arm until the break falls (back) into place. Then two splints of linen are made and applied to the inside and underside of the arm'. The linen was then bound with a substance that hardened and was kept in place until the fracture healed. This simple splinting of a fracture was successful and the stiffener may have been asphalt or pitch brought from Saba in what is now the Yemen.[1] Fractures of the ulna have been studied in more than 100 bones from this time, with satisfactory alignment following splinting and only one showed signs of sepsis. It is probable that these were all closed fractures, as compound fractures where the skin is broken and the bone exposed usually became septic and the sufferer died.

Reference:

1. Science and Secrets of Early Medicine. By Jurgen Thorwald. Translated from the German by Richard and Clara Winston. Thames and Hudson Ltd. 1962, p 72.

Reduction of a dislocated jaw. (Edwin Smith Papyrus).

Also, in the papyrus is the following description concerning a dislocation. 'If you examine a man having a dislocation of his mandible, should you find his mouth open, and his mouth cannot close again, you should put your two thumbs upon the ends of the two rami of the mandible inside his mouth and your fingers under his chin and you should cause them to fall back, so they rest in their places'.[1] Practical descriptions of physical examination, diagnosis and treatment were given without incantations except in one case.

Failure of a treatment administered could result in punishment.[2]

In about 400 BC, Hippocrates (c460–377 BC) produced the first great surgical treatise on fractures. He described in detail, fractures of all the bones of the body. The setting and splinting of bones in the natural position and the expected length of time for healing to occur. He also described atrophy of muscles and understood the dangers of necrosis.[3] Management for the reduction of a dislocated mandible was similar to that given in the Smith Papyrus. Aulus Cornelius Celsus (c25 BC–c50 AD), four hundred years after Hippocrates, produced an encyclopaedia, *De Medicina*, that was used as a primary source on medicine and surgery until the sixteenth century. In it, he names many anatomical structures and his descriptions of the management of fractures builds on the work of Hippocrates with which he was familiar,[4] so demonstrating the continuity of practice.

References:

1. *The Healing Hand. Man and Wound in the Ancient World.* By Guido Majno. Harvard University Press 1985.
2. *A History of Surgery.* By Harold Ellis. Published by Greenwich Medical Media Ltd. 2001. ISBN 1 84110 023 4.
3. *Hippocratic Writings in Penguin Classics.* Edited by G.E.R. Lloyd, Translated by J. Chadwick and W.N. Mann, 1950 reprinted 1983. Pages 279–314.
4. *Celsus on Medicine, Book 8.* Translated by W.G. Spencer. Loeb Classical Library, Harvard University Press. First Published in 1938.

Use of sutures to close wounds. (Edwin Smith Papyrus).

Among original procedures was the closing of wounds of the lips, throat and shoulder with sutures. There is no information of what the suture material was made.[1] Also described are adhesive plasters that were used to draw the lips of a wound together, these were made from strips of linen, always in pairs with tree resin as the adhesive. This was commonly used when wounds were infected and sutures would not hold. Dr Guido Majno noted that taping wounds became commonplace in the 1800s in Europe when sepsis was endemic and many died from sepsis.[2]

References:

1. *Edwin Smith Surgical Papyrus.* By James Henry Breasted. Published in Facsimile with translation and Commentary. University of Chicago Press, 1980.

2. *The Healing Hand.* By Guido Majno. Harvard University Press. 1985, paperback edition 1991.

The first use of cautery. (Edwin Smith Papyrus).

When dealing with bleeding blood-vessels in Ancient Egypt (c1,550 BC) the surgeon advised that, 'The knife should be heated in the fire', as cautery could stop the bleeding. He also suggested that cutting and burning at the same time, with a red-hot knife, might check bleeding.[1]

Hippocrates (460–370 BC) also used cautery liberally. For example, he used it to treat haemorrhoids. More boldly, he attempted to prevent recurrent subluxation of the shoulder joint by using cautery. The idea was to hold the joint in place by cutting parallel incisions in the armpit with a red-hot knife to cause skin contraction,[2] hoping that this would hold the shoulder in place. He was careful to avoid the neurovascular tissues in the axilla.[3] Its success in curing the dislocation is not mentioned, but must have failed and been extremely painful.

In 1908, a technique to stop bleeding from small blood vessels during an operation was introduced by Carl Franz Nagelschmitd (1875–1952) who coined the word diathermy. He carried out extensive experiments on patients using diathermy and published the first textbook on the subject in 1913. Surgical diathermy, or electrocautery, involves the use of high frequency electric current as either a cutting tool or to coagulate small vessels that were bleeding has remained an essential surgical instrument ever since.[4]

References:

1. *Edwin Smith Surgical Papyrus.* By James Henry Breasted. Published in Facsimile with translation and Commentary. University of Chicago Press, 1980.
2. *Hippocrates Vol VIII. Loeb Classical Library.* Edited by Paul Potter. Harvard University Press, 1995.
3. *The Healing Hand.* By Guido Majno. Harvard University Press. Paperback Edition, 1991, p. 165.
4. Wikipedia. Diathermy.

c1,700 BC. Ancient Egypt. Incision of abscesses.

These is evidence in the Eber's Papyrus that Ancient Egyptians incised and drained abscesses at about this time.

A mass of tablets written in cuneiform were discovered in the former library of the destroyed palace of Assurbanipal, the palace of the last great king of Assyria. Twenty thousand tablets were excavated and amongst those of most recent date were a few tablets related to surgery. One describes the incision of a scalp abscess,[1] for infections and abscesses have always been common.

Reference:

1. *The Healing Hand.* By Guido Majno. Harvard University Press. 1985, paperback edition 1991.

c1,550 BC Ancient Egypt. The use of antiseptics.

Malachite, a green stone composed of copper carbonate was used over millennia by Egyptian women as a cosmetic for their eyes. Malachite has a powerful antibacterial effect and probably warded off the common eye diseases of the near east. Copper was also prepared as Verdigris and then applied to wounds as a poultice. The ancient Egyptians often added dung or ground flies to their mixture, making their treatment positively dangerous. In the same document, a salve of honey and grease was also in common use. This demonstrates that there was no clear-cut distinction at that time between magic and empiricism. The use of antiseptics in Egypt has been studied, tested and described by Dr Guido Majno.[1] The Egyptian rationale for adding foul substances to place in wounds is explained in Chapter 7.

Reference:

1. *The Healing Hand.* By Guido Majno. Harvard University Press. 1985, Paperback Edition 1991. Pages 111–120.

Chapter 4
Analysis of Surgery in the First Period
10,000 BC to 700 BC

1. Peru, the first operation.
2. The Ancient Egyptians develop the basic surgical procedures.
3. Differentiation of an original operation from later modifications and improvements.

1. Peru, the first operation.

The discovery of trephines in skulls from ancient Peru and elsewhere has already been discussed.[1] The rationale for the gradual spread of trephination across continents over millennia has been explained by Dr P. Piroschki (1930–2014) who observed that 10% of all skulls discovered from Neolithic times were trephined.

What Piroschki also noticed was some of these trephines had been started but not completed. He suggested that this may have been due to an unconscious man who had suffered a head injury, most likely in battle, had woken up while his skull was being trephined. It seems reasonable to speculate that they knew from experience that people who received penetrating wounds to the thorax or abdomen died. However, some with head injuries who appeared dead could be saved and regain consciousness following trephination. Unknown to the Peruvians, a beneficial but incidental consequence of opening the skull would be to release pressure on the brain if a blood clot had formed in the space between the skull and the dura mater, the strong membrane covering the brain. The ancient Peruvians believed in evil spirits, in which case the purpose of trephining the skull was magical with the objective of setting them free. If successful, the trephine would result in the 'dead' being awakened.

Piroschki's explanation[2] suggests that Neolithic surgeons protected the brain by releasing pressure on the brain in these circumstances would cause the person to regain consciousness. In effect, the 'dead' would come back to life once the 'evil spirits had escaped'. This must have occurred quite frequently judging from the fact that many of the skulls had more than one trephine with its associated fracture[3] from earlier conflicts.

The first written description of this operation was a brief account by Hippocrates (460–370 BC).[4] Later, Aulus Celsus (c25 BC–c50 AD),[5] a Roman encyclopaedist, provided a lucid description of the operation with significant technical improvements. These included a drill to cut through the skull which is the prototype of the instrument used today. He also described a new technique to extend the operation by raising a cranial flap to gain better access to a site of haemorrhage. The Greek approach to trephination of the skull was therefore rational and aimed at releasing pressure on the brain either from a blood clot or a depressed fracture. This is a demonstration of how an original operation was subsequently rationalised, modified and improved over time.

Another unexpected discovery from ancient Peru was that very few of the skulls showed any signs of post-operative infection. Neither Thomas Gale (1507–1587)[6] in England in the 16th century or Richard Wiseman[7] (1622–1676) in the 17th century mention post-operative sepsis following trephination in their books. This was not to last, for by the first half of the 19th century in Europe the results of trephination were disastrous as nearly all patients died from postoperative sepsis. This was so serious that trephination was abandoned and only reintroduced after the introduction of operating using the antiseptic surgery technique devised by Joseph Lister in 1865.[8]

The explanation for Gale and Wiseman's trephines having a lower fatality due to sepsis may have been due to fewer pathogenic bacteria on battlefields than in the unhygienic cities of Europe. This was before the cause of sepsis was understood, when the streets were also sewers. It was only in 1866 that London was connected to its first sewage network. Perhaps, there is an omen for 21st century surgeons if antibiotic resistant bacteria cannot be controlled.[9]

2. The Ancient Egyptians develop the basic surgical procedures.

The Ancient Egyptians produced six original operations and procedures over a period of 1,500 years. The first took place about 7,000 years after the Peruvian operation. These original-procedures were catheterisation[10] of the bladder carried out by passing a tube of vegetable origin into the bladder via the urethra, the splinting of fractures and reductions of dislocations,[11] the use of sutures[12] to close wounds and cautery to stop bleeding.[13] There was only two original operations, circumcision[14] probably the first elective or planned operation to be performed on a human, although it is uncertain whether it was initially for ritual or hygienic reasons. The other operation was to drain abscesses by incision, as described by the Ancient Egyptians.

The reason for enumerating the operations and procedures of the Ancient Egyptians is to draw attention not only to the simplicity of their surgery, but also that it was they who developed the foundation procedures of surgery that are still practiced today. This was the actual beginning of surgery and demonstrated what was possible at that time. With this in mind, the Peruvian operation when compared to these, might appear to be a complex procedure, but once learned is not a difficult operation to perform[15]. This is supported by the way it was copied and practiced across the Americas and Eurasia over millennia. Hippocrates' use of trephination to release pressure on the brain was entirely rational.

The Ancient Egyptians were the first to begin to formulate a theory of disease. Capable as they were of great engineering feats such as building the pyramids, they were also superstitious and believed in magic. This over a long period of time began to be rationalised and as a result turned into the practice of medicine. How this happened has been deduced from two ancient medical papyri. Both of these have been dated to around 1,700 BC. The contents of the *Eber's papyrus*[16] were medical and magical throughout, while the Edwin Smith Papyrus is almost completely rational and surgical. The *Eber's papyrus* consists of a collection of prescriptions that relate to the stomach, the heart and its blood vessels, where symptoms are described and interspersed with magical texts and incantations. The *Smith Papyrus* is concerned with the treatment of wounds and bone fractures described in forty-eight individual surgical cases. However, it does not entirely escape medico-magical incantations that are mentioned on 13 occasions.

Unfortunately, the *Smith Papyrus* is incomplete, descriptions of surgical treatment to the lower half of the body were lost.

In general, magic played a prominent part in the social and religious life of the Ancient Egyptians. This involved not only their relationships with people both living and dead but also with their gods. Through magic, it was believed that the problems of life, especially injury and disease could be solved with the help of a powerful magician. The name of this magic was 'hîke', a mystical power that was soon personified as a god. By virtue of this, the magicians performed a complex series of rites that are magical. The services of a magician were commonly sought to cure a disease thought to be caused by some poison or evil inflicted on a person by a demon that had entered their body. This malign spirit could be a god or goddess, a dead person or a living enemy. Once in the body, the demon made the person ill and the role of the magician was to get rid of it by exorcism.

Initially, the magician would recite a spell in which the demon was ordered to leave or for the poison to flow from the inflicted person's body. These spells often referred to the gods and could be accompanied by a ritual. This was the oral rite. There was a second or manual rite that could be as simple as using a string of beads or the wearing of an amulet. More often though the manual rite could take the form of repeating a formula to exorcise the demon or to take a mixture of substances that were given to the sufferer to swallow. Many of these mixtures contained foul medicines including copro-therapy that were so disgusting that it was supposed to distress the possessing spirits, inducing them to leave the sufferer's body. One wonders how the patient felt, as the magician always had other similar remedies if the first failed.

Some of these secondary therapies contained drugs. The huge variety of prescriptions found in *Eber's medical papyrus* confirms their arbitrary and unscientific use. The numerous alternatives show that if one fails another formula was always available. Gradually, the magicians would recognise that some of their prescriptions were actually more helpful to the sufferer than others and began to prescribe these more frequently as medicines and not just to exorcise an evil spirit. As a result, they gradually came to place more faith in some drugs.

Slowly, over a long period of time, magicians began to abandon the magic and trust more in their treatments. Eventually, they became recognisable as physicians for 'Out of magic came medicine'.[17] For many, the magic continued as it always had. For throughout history, new discoveries or treatments did not ever completely displace the old ways, as shown by the continuing practice of magic in the Middle Ages some of which survives into modern times, including wearing of amulets to give a simple example. Surgery was not troubled by these problems, as the usefulness of its practice when successful was self-evident.

BOX 4.1

The first period of surgery with eight original operations and procedures.

c 10,000 BC	Peru	Operation of trephination of the skull[1].
c 3,000 BC	Egypt	Procedure of catheterisation.[10]
c 2,500 BC	Egypt	Operation of cimcumcision[14].
c 1,700 BC	Egypt	Procedure of splinting of fractures[11].
c 1,700 BC	Egypt	Procedure of reducing dislocations[11].
c 1,700 BC	Egypt	Procedure of suturing wounds[12].
c 1,700 BC	Egypt	Procedure of cautery[13].
c 1,700 BC	Egypt	Incision of abscesses[20].

Egyptian physicians became famous in the ancient world and were known to have specialised. Herodotus (c484-425 BC) extolled their virtues in treating the Kings of Persia,[18] not always with success. He describes when Darius (522–486 BC), King of Persia had fallen and seriously dislocated an ankle. He called his Egyptian Doctors who made the situation worse. He was informed by his servants that a Greek physician, Democedes of Crotona was skilled in these matters. Democedes was a prisoner having been captured by the Persians and was to be found among their slaves. He treated Darius successfully and was rewarded and released.

Connections between Egypt and Greece also involved trade. The Ancient Greeks had need of antiseptics such as nitron, a yellow crystalline precipitate of nitrate, also alum, perfumes, thread and leather and it is known that the Egyptians bought opium from the Greeks from as early as the 12th century BC.

Ancient Egyptians had little knowledge of anatomy, but through mummification knew a little bit about it. They named about a hundred parts of the body, especially the gut and heart. The heart was considered the most important organ and was preserved with the mummy while the brain was considered of less value and was removed. They had no understanding of the function of the nerves, muscles, arteries or veins. These latter were thought to be the conduits for blood, air, nutrition, water, mucus and other secretions. The rectum and anus were believed to be significant portals for disease to spread into the body.

The surgeon in the *Edwin Smith Papyrus* gave specific instructions of how to approach the treatment of a wounded patient. First, the patient was to be examined, then a diagnosis made and finally a prognosis is given. The prognosis is divided into three categories, expressed as follows, 'An ailment that I will treat', 'An ailment with which I will contend or wrestle with' and 'An ailment not to be treated'.

This approach to the injured and wounded was rational, although there was a hint that there might be an evil spirit, lurking in the phrase, to be 'wrestled with', that was included among the conditions with which the surgeon had announced he would contend. This could imply a belief in magic, for as previously noted the Smith papyrus does contain a few magical incantations in the text and on the back of the papyrus is written a collection of charms and prescriptions.[19] The habit of mummification of the pharaohs and nobles also broke a taboo that was thought to eventually lead to the acceptance of examining and dissecting the dead.

The Egyptians in the Ebers papyrus, c1,700 BC, described the incision of an abscess. Later, the Assyrians who developed a cuneiform form of writing using tablets of clay. First discovered in the 1800s after having laid hidden for over three thousand years in the pile of rubble that was once the fabled city of Nineveh. On one of these tablets was described instructions of how to incise an abscess on the scalp dating from c630 BC.[20] This was also the era of the first laws regulating surgery. Draconian punishments took place if a patient died, for these laws were carved in stone in Assyria at about the same time.

3. Another example differentiating an original operation from a successor surgeon's modifications and improvements.

The immobilisation of fractured bones was first described in the Smith Papyrus. The surgeon developed a paste, probably from tar or gum resin that set hard when mixed with linen and was used to hold the fracture in position to allow it to heal satisfactorily. The success of this has been confirmed by a collection of healed fractures found in an ossuary in Ancient Egypt. Assistants and pupils who helped to set fractures copied the method. This resulted in this treatment being passed on, knowing that the bone would unite in a satisfactory position. Gradually, the same technique was applied to suitable fractures elsewhere on the body. Copying these principles for treatment on other fractured bones in the body does not qualify them to be original procedures, as they are copying and applying an already known technique.

References:

1. Chapter 2. c10,000 BC. Trephination of skull.
2. A History of Medicine: primitive and ancient medicine. Piroschki P. Omaha, Nebraska: Horatius Press; 1995; p. 21–30.
3. Neolithic Trepanation decoded – A unifying hypothesis: Has the mystery as to why primitive surgeons performed cranial surgery been solved. Miguel A Faria. Surgical Neurology International. 2015: 6: 72. 2.
4. Chapter 2. c425 BC. Hippocrates
5. Ibid. c30.AD. Celsus.
6. Certaine Vvorkes of Chirurgerie. By Thomas Gale, 1507–1585, Hall Rowland, D. 1563, Printer. Nabu Public Domain Reprints.
7. Richard Wiseman. Several Chirurgical Treatises by Richard Wiseman (1686). London Printed by R. Norton and J. Macock, for R. Royston and B. Took. Henry E. Huntington Library and Art Gallery.
8. Chapter 2. 1865. Lord Lister.
9. Ibid. 1929. Antibiotic resistance.
10. Ibid. c3,000 BC. Catheterisation.
11. Ibid. c1,700 BC. Dislocations and fractures.
12. Ibid. c1,700 BC. Sutures. Paragraph 3.
13. Ibid. c10,000 BC. Cautery.
14. Ibid. c2,500 BC. Circumcision.
15. The End of the Golden Age of General surgery. 1870–2000. By N. K. Maybury. ISBN 1499531370. CreateSpace Independent Publishing Platform, North Charleston, South Carolina. p 28.
16. Chapter 2. 1,550 BC. Ebers Papyrus.
17. Egypt's place in Medical History, Science, Medicine and History. Essays on the Evolution of Scientific Thought and Medical Practice. Written in Honour of Charles Singer. Volume One. By E Ashworth, Edited by E. A. Underwood. Oxford University Press. 1953. Egypt's Place in Medical History by Warren R. Dawson. P. 47–60.
18. Herodotus. The Histories. Penguin Classics. Revised Edition 1982. P. 204.
19. The Edwin Smith Surgical papyrus, Volume 1. Published in Facsimile and Hieroglyphic Transliteration with Translation and Commentary in

Two Volumes. Volume One by James Henry Breasted. The University of Chicago Press, Chicago, USA.
20. Chapter 2. c1,700 BC. Incision of abscesses.

Chapter 5: Second Period
699 BC To 641 AD.
Ancient Greece, Rome and India

Original Operation in Ancient Greece, Rome and India with Subsequent Developments

c425 BC Greece. Hippocrates of Cos and the beginning of rational medicine.

Hippocrates (460–370 BC) kept records of his patients. This enabled him to diagnose a patient's disease from their signs and symptoms and so give them an accurate prognosis. He could then tell the patient precisely what their symptoms had been from the onset of the disease. This would have impressed them. If his prognosis indicated that the patient would not survive, he would not treat them. It is possible that in these cases he would 'refer' the patient to a Temple of Aesculapius.

The descriptions of his original operations have survived, having been copied many times and passed through multiple translations. Some of the operations he described may have been performed by un-named Greek surgeons before he described them.[1] Since their names are unknown, all these operations have been attributed to Hippocrates for simplicity.

He was the first to understand and teach that all diseases had natural causes and were not due to the displeasure of the gods. His original operations are described below. He also practised operations and procedures that were legacies from Peru and Ancient Egypt, for example, he considerably expanded the knowledge of how to manage fractures and dislocations. Below are listed his original operations.

Reference:

1. *Hippocratic writings*. Edited by Sir Geoffrey Lloyd, translated by J.

Chadwick and W.N. Mann. Penguin Classics 1950, reprinted 1983.

Fistula-in-ano.

This was an original operation by Hippocrates, whose instructions for treating an anal fistula were as follows. 'Take a span of very fine thread of raw linen, fold it in five, twist it together and wrap it around a horsehair'. Then pass the 'thread through the eye of a probe made of soft tin. Insert the probe into the fistula and with a finger of the other hand in the anus guide it through the internal opening of the fistula. Remove the probe and then tie the ends of the thread. Any slackness in the thread should be tightened daily. If the thread dissolves before the fistula is eaten through, replace it'. Hippocrates then covered the wound with an antiseptic, in this case using burned flower of copper.[1]

According to Hippocrates, riding and rowing were the commonest professions that led to the development of fistula-in-ano. His description of the operation would not be out of place in a modern textbook of surgery.

Fistula-in-ano begins as an abscess in an anal gland, that instead of discharging into the rectum discharges through the skin outside at the side of the anus. This leaves a track from the internal opening of the anal gland to the skin, and because it runs outside the muscle of the anal sphincter, it will continue to leak faeces indefinitely until skilfully operated upon.

Four hundred years later, Aulus Cornelius Celsus (c25 BC–c50 AD), a Roman encyclopaedist and surgeon, describes fistulae of the chest wall, abdomen as well as the anus.[2] All were secondary to internal infections that developed into abscesses that then discharged through the skin to cause a fistulous tract. Celsus' description for treating a fistula-in-ano was identical to that of Hippocrates. The seton (tie) slowly cuts through the anal muscle following its regular tightening. This causes fibrosis, stiffness of the sphincter muscle that maintains the integrity of the sphincter and so preserves continence. This is the operation still practiced today.

Treatment for fistula-in-ano was later recorded in Muslim Spain in the 11th century by al-Hashimi, who also described haemorrhoidectomy,[3] another of Hippocrates' original operations.

The first European description and treatment of fistula-in-ano was by John of Arderne (1306–1390), an English surgeon who was thought to be the first to devise some surgical cures including the operation for fistula-in-ano and has been regarded as the father of surgery in England, as noted in Chapter 1. At that time, it was not known that he had attended the University of Montpellier, the first Western European University to also have a Medical School, founded in 1160. There, Arderne had access to the surgical treatises of both Hippocrates and Galen, including Hippocrates' surgical treatment for fistula-in-ano. These had been translated from Greek into Arabic in Baghdad, and then into Latin by Constantine the African (c1020–1087) in Salerno in Italy. These translations were widely disseminated in Italy and later, France and would have therefore been available to Arderne.

Arderne declared that a peri-anal abscess must be lanced speedily to prevent it bursting into the rectum, 'or else, forsooth, it will burst within the anus…and if it bursts within and without (the anus), it can never be cured without a surgeon, full expert in his craft'. Arderne's operating technique was identical to that of Hippocrates and Celsus. The original operation therefore remains attributed to Hippocrates. Arderne practiced as a military surgeon[4] and most of his fistula-in-ano patients were from the nobility, who spent lengthy periods of time riding in armour, alternating between sweating profusely and freezing.

References:

1. Hippocrates Volume VIII. Edited and translated by Paul Potter. Loeb Classical Library. Harvard University press 1995 p. 387.
2. *Celsus on Medicine. Book VII.* Translated by W.G. Spencer. First published 1938 by Loeb Classical Library. ISBN 988-0-674-99370-9.
3. *Medieval Islamic Medicine.* Peter E. Pormann & Emily Savage Smith. Edinburgh University Press. 2010. ISBN 988 0 7486 2066 1, p. 130.
4. *A History of Surgery* by Harold Ellis. Greenwich Medical Media Ltd. 2001.

Haemorrhoidectomy.

Hippocrates, in the 5th century BC gives a contemporary description of his theory of haemorrhoids. He wrote, 'The condition arises when bile or phlegm becomes fixed in the vessels of the anus, it heats the blood in them so that being heated, they attract blood from their neighbours. As the (blood) vessels fill up, the interior of the anus becomes prominent and the heads of the vessels are raised above its surface, where they are partly abraded by the faeces passing out, and partly overcome by the blood collected inside them, and so spurt out blood, usually at defecation, but occasionally at other times as well'.

Hippocrates' original operation was to burn the haemorrhoids by cautery with a red-hot iron. Assistants were needed to hold the patient down during the operation. He states that bandages needed to be used for 20 days post-operatively.[1] His description has the feel of a practising surgeon who is familiar with haemorrhoids, even if his theory of the disease is wrong. This was an original operation by Hippocrates. The theory of the disease could have come from the Ancient Egyptians with their imaginary extensive plexus of blood vessels internal to the anus that were thought to be a principle source of disease in the body.[2]

Sir Frederick Treves' in his *Manual of Operative Surgery,* published in 1910, describes three different operations for treating haemorrhoids. These include ligating them, crushing them or using cautery to burn them. He noted that it is impossible to select one of these as the best.[3]

The modern operation for 3rd and 4th degree haemorrhoids is ligation and excision. First and 2nd degree haemorrhoids are usually injected or constricted by rubber bands.[4] In the 1980s, there was a brief vogue for treating haemorrhoids through freezing them by cryotherapy. This operation was rapidly abandoned as freezing has the same deleterious effect as the cautery used by Hippocrates. For when either of these methods were used, the tissues deep to the haemorrhoids are to a greater or lesser extent burnt or frozen. The result from either of these treatments was for the wound to weep post operatively for about 20 days, just as Hippocrates described when he used cautery. Both these techniques have since been abandoned.

References:

1. *Hippocrates. Volume VIII.* Edited and translated by Paul Potter. Loeb Classical Library. Harvard University Press, 1995.
2. Chapter 6.
3. *A manual of Operative Surgery.* Vol. 2. By Frederick Treaves 1892. Republished by Forgotten Books. ISBN 988-1-330-27819-2.
4. *General Surgery Lecture Notes.* By Harold Ellis, Sir Roy Calne, Christopher Watson. Wiley Blackwell, 2011.

Excision of a dead foetus at term.

Hippocrates describes in detail how to remove a dead foetus vaginally, with the safety and preservation of the mother in mind. This would be for a foetus at term as earlier in pregnancy such a foetus would usually be aborted spontaneously.

Reference:

1. *Hippocrates Volume IX.* Edited and translated by Paul Potter. Loeb Classical Library. Harvard University Press. 2010.

The Operation of Venesection.

For millennia, the Ancient Egyptians had a theory that the pus produced in most wounds was associated with bad blood. The persistence of this idea led Hippocrates to reason that it was possible to drain the 'bad' blood[1] by opening the vein nearest to the infection with a scalpel. On another occasion, he advised that a person with a violent nosebleed should also undergo venesection.[2.] Aulus Cornelius Celsus (c30 AD) in Rome also recorded the liberal use of bleeding patients.[3]

As a treatment, it is completely useless and often harmful, even so it was still being practised into the 19th century when the use of leeches became the favoured way to bleed patients. Leeches are still used in some places to this day. The theory from which venesection developed is described in Chapter 7.

References:

1. *The Healing Hand. Man and Wound in the Ancient World.* By Guido Majno. Harvard University Press. Paperback Edition 1991.
2. *Hippocrates Volume VIII.* Edited and translated by Paul Potter. Loeb Classical Library. Harvard University Press. 1995.
3. *Celsus on Medicine Book 3.* Translated by W.G. Spencer. Loeb Classical Library. Harvard University Press. 1935. P. 395.

Excision of bladder stones.

The fist reference to 'cutting for the stone' is mentioned by Hippocrates in his 'Oath' and dates from before 425 BC. In this book, the original operation for excising a bladder stone through a perineal incision has been attributed to Hippocrates.[1] Although he did not carry out the operation himself it was then being practiced in Greece by families of itinerant 'cutters for the stone'. This mention by Hippocrates is now thought to predate Sushruta,[2] the famous Indian surgeon's book *The Sushruta Samhita* by about 200 years[3]. The difficulty here has been to match the dates of the 'oral' Indian tradition, in which dates are not recorded, with those of the Ancient Greek treatises.

Aulus Cornelius Celsus[4] gives a detailed and coherent description of the operation which is briefly summarised here. The patient must be kept still so the surgeon could operate and this required four strong men as assistants. Two to hold the patient's legs and press down with their chests on his shoulders to keep him still and two others to ensure that these men did not slip as they would not be able to let go and adjust themselves. The surgeon after preparing himself gently introduced two fingers of the left hand into the anus and the right hand on the abdomen to gently push the stone into the pelvis where it could be held in place by the fingers of the left hand. He then made an inverted semilunar incision above the anus and then opened the neck of the bladder and delivered the stone.

This operation had been practised from the 4th century BC with a mortality of about 50%. Not surprisingly, its reputation[5] was bad but the pain caused by bladder stones was so excruciating that it drove patients to seek treatment. The main complications from which patients died were bleeding and sepsis.

This perineal approach for removal a bladder stone was later attributed to Jacques de Beaulieu in about 1700 as an original operation. This attribution was wrong, for long ago it had been practiced in Ancient Greece and India as described above.[6] Celsus' Latin manuscript, *De Medicina,* includes a description of this operation that had been available in the universities of Europe from the 15th century.[7]

Jean Civiale (1792–1867) of Paris in 1824 made an instrument that he called a 'trilabe'. This was introduced through the urethra to grasp, break and remove bladder stones.[8] Before this, Sushruta's[5] operation had been carried out on Samuel Pepys (1633–1703) the London Diarist in March 1658. Pepys was so happy to have survived that afterwards, he celebrated every year on the anniversary of the operation[9].

Following the introduction of anaesthesia, the perineal approach was abandoned and replaced by an abdominal approach to open the bladder and remove stones.

References:

1. *Cutting for stone: the ancient art of lithotomy.* Harry H. Herr. Dept Urol. Memorial Sloan-Kettering Cancer Centre, Weill-Cornell Medical College, NY, NY. Onlinelibrary.wiley.com 15 Nov 2007.
2. *A History of Medicine. Volume II. Early Greek, Hindu and Persian Medicine.* By Henry E. Sigerist. Oxford University Press 1961. ISBN 988-0-19-505079-0. P 182.
3. Menon I.A., Haberman H.F. 1969. Dermatological writings of ancient India. Med. Hist. 13(4): 387–392.
4. *Celsus on Medicine. III, Loeb Classical Library. Book 7.* Translated by W.G. Spencer. Harvard University Press, Cambridge Massachusetts London, England. p 431–441.
5. *Hippocratic Writings.* By G.E.R. Lloyd. Penguin Classics, reprinted 1983. And, *The Diaries of Samuel Pepys.* Edited by Robert Latham. Penguin Classics. Reprint 2003.
6. *The Healing Hand.* By Guido Majno. Harvard University Press. 1985, paperback edition 1991.
7. *Arabian Medicine and its influence on the Middle Ages. Vol 1.* By Dr Donald Campbell. 1926. London. Kegan Paul, Trench, Trubner & Co., Ltd. Broadway House, Charter Lane, London. p 177.
8. *The Diary of Samuel Pepys.* By Robert Latham. Published by Bell and Hyman, 1985.
9. *Medicine, Cambridge Illustrated History.* Edited by Roy Porter. Published by the Press Syndicate of the University of Cambridge. 1996. ISBN 0-521-44211-7. P. 219.

c320 BC India. The first birth by Caesarean section.

The earliest recorded birth by 'Caesarean' section was of Bindusara (c320–c272 BC), who became the second Mauryan Emperor of India.[1] A caesarean section in antiquity could only have taken place in the palace of a King, as it would be essential for a skilled surgeon to be in attendance at the childbirth with immediate access to suitable instruments.

The claim that Julius Caesar (100–44 BC) was born by caesarean section is untrue. His mother, Aurelia Cotta, was born in 120 BC and gave birth to Caesar in 100 BC when she was twenty. She died in 54 BC at the age of 66. There are no records of a mother surviving the operation in classical times[2] and when the operation was carried out, it was usually an attempt to save an important heir.

In the 1990s, an English consultant obstetrician carried out an emergency post mortem caesarean-section. This was done to deliver a baby in circumstances where the mother had suffered a cardiac arrest. An emergency caesarean section can be carried out in sixty seconds. So, the decision to operate needs to be taken within four minutes of the mother's cardiac arrest. This gives just enough time for the baby to be delivered in under five minutes after the mother's heart had stopped beating and the baby is no longer being oxygenated. If delivered within five minutes, the chances of the baby suffering brain damage due to lack of oxygen is significantly reduced. Another caveat is that the baby should be 37 weeks or more. In modern times, such a delivery has achieved the baby's survival without brain damage in 70% of them.

The case quoted here took place in the Accident and Emergency department of a District General Hospital. The consultant obstetrician was in his outpatient clinic at the time. The mother who was already in labour had been brought into the Accident & Emergency Department having had two eclamptic fits and her ECG was showing ventricular fibrillation. On arrival at the hospital, she had a cardiac arrest. The consultant obstetrician was immediately called and reached the A&E Department in under three minutes of her arrival. He instantly decided to carry out a section. The baby was near term and survived normally. Every effort was made to resuscitate the mother but this was unsuccessful.[3]

References:

1. Lurie S. (2005). The changing motives of caesarean section from the ancient world to the twenty-first century. Archives of Gynaecology and Obstetrics. Springer. 271 (4): 281–285.
2. Wikipedia. Julius Caesar.
3. Personal communication 2017.

c260 BC Greece. Herophilos of Chalcedon. Anatomy and the first human dissections.

Herophilos (335–280 BC) was a great anatomist at the Museum and Library in Alexandria in Egypt. He was permitted to carry out dissections on condemned criminals during the reign of Ptolemy II Philadelphus (285–246 BC), there is no evidence that human vivisection was permitted elsewhere in the Greek world or contemplated anywhere thereafter.

Herophilos considered it essential to base knowledge on an empirical basis and was the first to propose that the brain rather than the heart was the seat of the intellect. Due to his dissections, he is credited with having discovered the connection between the brain and the spinal cord and established the anatomical distinction between the arteries and veins, recognising that the blood vessel leading from the right ventricle to the lung was an artery and not a vein. He also named parts of the body with specific names, such as the duodenum.

Herophilos' works were lost, but he was extensively quoted by Galen of Pergamon (129–199 AD), who was himself a brilliant anatomist, lecturer and surgeon who practiced in Rome. After Galen, the Dark Ages descended and anatomy was not systematically studied for another 1300 years. It was rekindled by Vesalius (1514–1564) who published a new anatomy textbook in 1543. Herophilos was a contemporary of Erasistratus, who is described in the next entry.

Reference:

The Heart and Vascular System in Ancient Greek Medicine, from Alcmaeon to Galen. By C.R.S. Harris, Oxford at the Clarendon Press, 1983. P 178–181.

c260 BC Greece. Erasistratus of Ceos. The heart recognised as a one-way pump.

Erasistratus (c304–c250 BC) was a Greek physician in Alexandria, Egypt, who studied at the Museum during the reigns of early members of the Ptolemaic dynasty. He advanced anatomical knowledge through human dissection and was the first to understand the heart as a one-way pump, recognising the cardiac valves would only permit flow in one direction. Despite this, the role of the heart and lungs was not then understood.

Aristotle, (384–322 BC) believed that the heart was the seat of intelligence, while Erasistratus was the first to believe that it was the brain.[1] He was a contemporary of Herophilos.[2]

Ibn al-Nafīs (1213–1288) was the first to describe the flow of blood from the right ventricle of the heart to the lungs and then to the left ventricle, a significant advance. He did not make the connection with the greater circulation throughout the body.[3]

The circulation of the blood was to remain unknown until it was proved by Dr William Harvey[4] (1588–1658) following his observations and detailed research, published in 1628. Among his experiments, he measured the output of blood from an animal's heart and calculated that in a day the heart's output exceeded the volume of blood in the body many times over. The only conclusion was that blood must circulate in the body. This was before the capillaries were identified. Harvey's publication of a description of the circulation was nearly 1000 years after Erasistratus carried out his studies.

References:

1. *Greek science after Aristotle.* By G.E.R. Lloyd. Published by W.W. Norton & Company in 1983.
2. Wikipedia. Ibn al-Nafīs, and How Islam changed the world. Majeed Azeem (2005). BMJ 331 (7531): p 1486–1288.
3. Chapter 2, c260 BC
4. *The Anatomical Exercises. De Motu Cordis and De Circulatione Sanguinis.* In English Translation by William Harvey. Edited by Geoffrey Keynes. Dover Publications, Inc New York. 1953, republished 1995. ISBN.13: 988-0-486-68827-5.

c250 BC Greek. Ctesibius of Alexandria. Advances in technology, the invention of the syringe and pump.

The concept of a piston and cylinder forming a syringe, was developed in Alexandria in Egypt by Ctesibius, (c285–222 BC). It was used for injecting liquids and sucking out pus from wounds and abscesses.[1] He also invented the valve and because of this the pump. He was one of the greatest engineers of antiquity. His work was reported by the Roman architect, Marcus Vitruvius 250 years later. Ctesibus's inventions have been used ever since.[2]

References:

1. *The Heart and Vascular System in Ancient Greek Medicine, from Alcmaeon to Galen.* By CR.S. Harris, Oxford at the Clarendon Press, 1983.
2. Wikipedia. Ctesibius of Alexandria.

c200 BC India. Sushruta.

Sushruta (c200 BC) was a famous Hindu physician and author of a treatise on medicine and surgery. When it was written is uncertain and scholars in the past have given it a wide range of dates. The most recent study estimates the date of Sushruta's writing to be between 200 and 100 BC.[1 & 2] It is difficult to date his work because of the ancient Hindu tradition of passing on knowledge through an oral tradition. It has not been possible within a wide range of error to know when he lived. Some of the original operations recorded by Sushruta may have been carried out a century or more earlier, as illustrated for example by the date given for the treatment of snakebites inflicted on Alexander the Great's soldiers when he invaded India in 327 BC.

The text of Sushruta's work was translated into Arabic by Kitab Shah Shun al-Hindi[3] in Baghdad early in the 8th century AD and reached Europe in the Medieval period. This can be considered another example of the dissemination of surgical knowledge and continuity in the practice of surgery.

References:

1. Menon I.A., Haberman H.F. 1969. Dermatological writings of ancient India. Med Hist. 13 (4): 387–392.
2. *Medival and Islamic Medicine.* By Peter E. Pormann and Emile Savage-Smith. In the New Edinburgh Islamic Surveys. Edinburgh University Press. ISBN 978 0 7486 2067 8. 1988, p 21–22.
3. *Encyclopaedia of Indian medicine*. By Ramachandra S.K. – Google Books.

Snakebites, the first use of a tourniquet.

Snakebites were and are frequent in India. Sushruta treated a person bitten on a limb with a tourniquet applied above the bite. An attempt was then made to suck the venom from the wound, followed by an incision between the fang marks with a sharp knife. Finally, if available, a concoction of 'sarpagandha' was taken by mouth.[1] This is the root of 'Rauwolfia serpentine', the Latin name for the source of the tranquilising drug Reserpine developed in the 1950s.

This use of a tourniquet followed by an incision for snakebites was known in 327 BC when Alexander the Great crossed the Indus. He unexpectedly found that many of his troops were bitten by cobras. Because the Greek physicians had no experience of this problem, Alexander hired Hindu physicians to treat those who had been bitten.

In 2015, Nature Journal of Science records that there were 100,000 people fatally bitten by poisonous snakes in a year. This was mainly in India, South-East Asia and Africa.[2]

A more general use of tourniquets to stop blood loss following serious wounds to the limbs does not seem to have been known in the Greek or Roman eras. In Europe in 1674, Etienne Morel, a military surgeon, used a tourniquet at the Battle of Flanders in France. Gradually thereafter, it was used to temporarily control severe limb haemorrhage. The opposing armies in the American Civil War used tourniquets and they have been used in all wars since[3].

References:

1. *The healing Hand.* By Guido Majno. Harvard University Press. 1985, paperback edition 1991. P 278–285.
2. Nature Journal of Science. 2017.
3. *A Brief History of the Tourniquet.* By D.R. Welling, P.L. McKay, T.E. Rosmuscan & M.M. Rich, www.jvascsurg.org

Origin of plastic surgery, earlobe reconstruction.

Sushruta wrote ten pages to describe earlobe piercing and its complications. The custom of enlarging an ear piercing to enable a heavy earring to be worn was favoured by the Brahmins of that era. Sometimes this resulted in sepsis or trauma causing the earlobe to be torn apart. Not being able to exhibit an earring was distressing and this complication of ear lobe piercing created a need for an enterprising surgeon to demonstrate his skill. This is an original operation and also the first plastic operation to be recorded.

Sushruta described a Brahmin whose earlobe had shrunk to a small scar after it was torn. He wrote, 'The ways to repair an injured earlobe are innumerable'. But, 'In this case, it can only be repaired by making a new earlobe out of the skin nearby. A surgeon well-versed in the knowledge of surgery should slice a patch of living flesh from the cheek of a person devoid of earlobes in a manner so as to have one of its ends (remain) attached to its former seat (on the cheek below the earlobe). Then the part where the artificial (new) earlobe is to be (attached), should be partly scarified with a knife and the living flesh, full of blood and sliced as previously directed, (the flap) should be 'adhesioned' to it'. Sushruta was the first to describe and create a pedicle flap.[1] Hindu surgeons were the pioneers of plastic surgery with this original operation.

It was Gaspar Tagliacozzi(1545–1599) an Italian surgeon in Bologna, who was regarded as the father of modern plastic surgery in Europe and raised it to new heights. He published: *On the Surgery of Mutilations by Grafting.* In this book, he describes years of trial and error, documented with drawings. He reconstructed ears, lips and noses.[2]

Nearly three hundred years later, Plastic Surgery became a surgical specialty and was further developed during World War One by Mr Harold Delf Gillies (1882–1960), a New Zealander in the Royal Army Medical Corps. A special unit was developed in Aldershot, England, where he used tube pedicle grafts to replace missing facial tissue and he also used bone grafts. His initial unit was overwhelmed due to the numbers of the wounded and a new 600-bed hospital bed was built in 1917. He had the advantage of general anaesthesia and was also dubbed the father of modern plastic surgery.[3]

The origin of the name 'plastic surgery' is from the Greek word *platikos* which means 'to mould' and such operations indicate that tissue is moved around in reconstructive operations.

References:

1. *The Healing Hand.* By Guido Majno. Harvard University Press. 1985, paperback edition 1991. 292–293.
2. *A History of Surgery.* By Harold Ellis. Greenwich Medical Media Ltd. 2001. And *The healing Hand.* By Guido Majno. Harvard University Press. 1985, paperback edition 1991. P 44.
3. British Journal of Plastic Surgery (1989), 32 68–77.

Plastic surgery. First nasal reconstruction.

In India, nasal reconstruction was uncommon, Sushruta devoted two pages to his technique for carrying this out and it is therefore an original operation. The new nose was formed by a pedicle flap of skin turned down while still attached to the forehead.[1] This work was translated into Arabic in about 800 by Rhazes.[2]

Disfigurement of the nose was caused by mutilation, trauma or syphilis. The graft was constructed from an arm flap.[3] Tagliacozzi's (1545-1599) operation does not qualify as an original operation as he uses a pedicle graft, albeit a sophisticated one, demonstrating an improvement in technique over that devised by Sushruta.

Reference:

1. *The Healing Hand.* By Guido Majno. Harvard University Press. 1985, paperback edition 1991. 288–291
2. *A History of Surgery.* By Harold Ellis. Publisher Greenwich Medical Media Ltd 2001. ISBN: 1-84110-023-4. P 44.

Couching of cataracts.

Sushruta devotes a chapter to couching cataracts. He used a needle, or fine lancet that was inserted behind the iris from above to mobilise the lens and then push it downwards, so it rested below the line of vision.[1] This is thought to be the first detailed description of this operation. However, there is a claim that it could have occurred much earlier in Mesopotamia but the interpretation of what was written is not clear and the primitive state of surgery at that time makes it very unlikely.[2] There was another speculation that couching of cataracts predates Sushruta and goes back to the 5th Dynasty in Egypt (c2,467–2,458 BC). This can also be dismissed as 800 years later, Egyptian surgery, as described in the *Smith Papyrus* written in about 1,700 BC describes surgery at a very elementary stage and was not then sophisticated enough to undertake couching of cataracts.[3]

In 1748, Dr Jacques Daviel[4](1696–1762), a French doctor was the first to extract a cataract from the eye in Europe. John Hunter (1728–1793) a famous surgeon in London of Scottish origin, describes in his *Lecture Notes of 1785*, 'I have seen suppuration take place in the eye three times after extraction of the crystalline lens, the posterior chamber (of the eye) being exposed'.[5]

The extraction of the lens is not considered an original operation as the technique of safely mobilising opaque lenses had already been demonstrated.

References:

1. *Sushruta Samhita.* Translated by K.L. Bhishagratna. Chowkhamba Sanskrit Series Office, Varanasi, India. Reprinted 1963. P 77–78.
2. *Science and Secrets of Early Medicine.* By Jurgen Thorwold. Published by Thames & Hudson, London 1962.
3. *Edwin Smith Papyrus.*
4. Wikipedia. Jacques Daviel. Extracapsular cataract extraction.
5. *Hunterian Reminiscences, being the Substance of a Course of Lectures on the Principles and Practice of Surgery Delivered by John Hunter in the Year 1785.* By James Parkinson. Published by Sherwood, Gilbert, and Piper, Paternoster Row. 1888. Reprinted Compton & Richie, Printer. 2019.

c30 AD. Rome. Aulus Cornelius Celsus.

Aulus Cornelius Celsus (c25 BC–c50 AD) produced an encyclopaedia, *De Medicina,* which was used as a primary textbook of medicine and surgery in Rome and Byzantium and was then lost until its rediscovery in the 1400s. Celsus was the most important surgical encyclopaedist in antiquity and his works were studied into the late medieval period. He lived four hundred years after Hippocrates of Cos (460–370 BC), and was followed one hundred and fifty years later by Galen of Pergamon (129–c200 AD).[1] His manuscripts, in common with those of Hippocrates, show evidence of including the operations of earlier surgeons, many of whom he names.[2] His work demonstrates a further advance in the understanding of anatomy and he described the original operations listed below. His publications were all in Latin, many of the surgeons he quotes were Greek, whose works he translated into Latin. This confirms the continuity of Greek operations into the Roman era.

He also named the four signs of inflammation as 'rubour, tumour, calour and dolour', that translates as redness, swelling, heat and pain. These were still taught in medical schools in the mid-twentieth century.

References:

1. *The Legacy of Rome.* Edited by Cyril Bailey. Oxford University Press. 1923, reprinted 1940.
2. *Celsus on Medicine Volume III, books 7–8.* Translated by W.G. Spencer, edited by Jeffery Henderson. Loeb Classical Library, Harvard University Press, 1938, p. 295–297.

Ligation of blood vessels.

Celsus wrote, 'When a man has been wounded who can be saved…he should not die from haemorrhage or inflammation'.[1] He went on to describe simple methods of treatment, such as pressure on the wound and the application of vinegar to stop the bleeding, but proceeded to say, 'The blood vessels which are pouring out blood are to be seized and a double ligature applied above the bleeding point'. His idea of applying a ligature to stop serious bleeding was a fundamental advance in emergency surgery and the first step towards what in the 20th century became vascular surgery.

Reference:

Celsus on Medicine, Volume II Book V. Translated by W.G. Spencer. Loeb Classical Library, Harvard University Press. ISBN 988-0-674-99335-8. 1938. p 403.

Amputation of limbs

Celsus (c25 BC–c50 AD) advised the amputation of gangrenous limbs. He recognised that this was 'not a safe option but is the only one in the circumstance'. He continued by writing, 'between the sound and the diseased part, the flesh is to be cut through with a scalpel to the bone'. He then directs that the joints should be avoided and that 'sound flesh should be cut away' (if necessary) to ensure that all diseased tissue is excised. The bone is then exposed well above the level of the skin incision before cutting through it with a saw, the rough parts of the bone are to be smoothed and the skin is drawn over it'.[1]

This technique for amputating a limb was used during the World War of 1914–1918. For when a bone stump following an amputation began to protrude through the skin, it was cut back to a higher level.

In earlier times, Hippocrates was aware of amputations, but was adept at managing gangrenous legs without doing so.[2] His principle was that under no circumstance should any living tissue be removed, for to do so could precipitate an extension of the area of gangrene, so he never sawed-off protruding bone, but waited for it to separate naturally which might take many months.

Francois Chopart (1743–1795) carried out an amputation of the forefoot at the mid tarsal joint and used the long flap of the sole of the foot to cover the stump.

References:

1. *Celsus on Medicine, Volume III Book VII.* Translated by W.G. Spencer. Loeb Classical Library, Harvard University Press. ISBN 988-0-674-99370-9. p 469–471.
2. *Hippocrates Vol. VIII.* Edited and translated by Paul Potter. Loeb Classical Library. Harvard University Press. 1995. P 345.
3. *A History of Surgery.* By Harold Ellis. Greenwich Medical Media Ltd. London. p 56.

Excision of tonsils

Tonsillectomy as described by Celsus (c25 BC–c50 AD) should be limited, 'to those that have a thin tunic around the tonsils following (chronic) inflammation and were (large enough to be) mobilised with a finger, then transfixed by a hook and excised with a scalpel'.[1] It seems that tonsils excised at that time were probably necrotic, otherwise torrential bleeding could occur that would be difficult to stop owing to the difficulty of reaching the bleeding vessels.

al-Zahrāwi, Abū al-Qāsim(f c1000 AD), also known as Albucasis, described an improvement in the technique of tonsillectomy. With the tongue held still by a tongue depressor, the swollen tonsil was lifted by a hook and then removed with a scissor like instrument with transverse blades, that both cut the tonsil and held it for removal from the throat. Then the patient had to gargle with water and vinegar and, if haemorrhage followed, a gargle with styptics was prescribed. Such procedures were quite within the surgical capabilities of the day.[2] A thousand years later, at the beginning of the 20th century, itinerant practitioners travelled in parts of the USA and Europe excising children's tonsils in their homes. They used virtually the same technique as described above.

References:

1. *Celsus on Medicine. Vol III Book VII.* Translated by W.G. Spencer. First published 1938 by Loeb Classical Library, Harvard University press. ISBN 988-0-674-99370-9. p 371–373.
2. *Medieval Islamic Medicine.* By Peter E. Pormann & Emily Savage Smith. Edinburgh University Press. 2010. ISBN 988 0 7486 2066 1. Page 64.

Umbilical hernias operation.

Celsus approached this operation by saying, 'No person would undergo surgery unless in severe pain and in danger of losing their life'. Then, 'In the case of an umbilical hernia, bowel and omentum may be found on opening the hernial sac and if the omentum is mortified (necrotic) it may fall off or must be cut away with shears (scissors) as bleeding will not occur'. Bleeding vessels were ligated and if the small bowel had prolapsed, it was pushed back into the abdomen. He continued, 'when the remaining omentum, if any, has been replaced the abdominal wall should be stitched'.[1]

Reference:

1. *Celsus on Medicine. Book VII.* Translated by W.G. Spencer. Loeb Classical Library, Harvard University Press 1935. ISBN 988-0-674-99322-8. P 377–381.

Inguinal hernia operation

With inguinal hernias, Celsus writes that 'if the omentum (has) comes down, the swelling in the scrotum never disappears, but if only the intestine comes down and is not inflamed, it can disappear (be pushed or slide back into the abdomen) when the patient is resting'.[1] An irreducible hernia may strangulate and present as a life-threatening situation, that can only be treated by surgery.

Celsus describes cutting down to the hernial sac which was excised. Post-operative bleeding was to be avoided by ligating blood vessels. After tying the knot, the ends of the ligatures were then left hanging out of the wound.[2] Such a wound not surprisingly always became infected, even so this remained the normal practice into the late Middle Ages. After a number of days, the surgeon would tug gently on the ligature and if the artery had healed, the ligature with its knot would slide out. If the artery had not healed and the ligature came away, severe bleeding could follow. This could be impossible to control, especially if it was from the leg, when the patient often bled to death.

In 1727, Rhamdohr successfully removed two feet of gangrenous bowel that had been incarcerated in an obstructed inguinal hernia. This was recorded in New York Med, Rec., Sept 22 1883.[3] The peritoneal cavity was not otherwise opened.

Reference:

1. *Celsus on Medicine. Book VII.* Translated by W.G. Spencer. Loeb Classical Library, Harvard University Press 1935. ISBN 988-0-674-99322-8. P. 379.
2. *Celsus on Medicine. Book VII.* Translated by W.G. Spencer. Loeb Classical Library, Harvard University Press 1935. ISBN 988-0-674-99322-8. p 381.
3. *A Manual of Operative Surgery. Vol. 2.* By Frederick Treves. Cassell & Company, Ltd: 1892, p 317.

Operation for varicocele

In this condition, Celsus wrote that when, 'The veins in the scrotum become swollen and twisted and massed together, they distend the scrotum generally and the testicle on that side hangs lower than it ought'. When operating, 'The groin is to be incised and the veins are to be separated and ligated'. He also notes that the operation scar can bind together the margins of the incision.

Reference:

1. *Celsus on Medicine.* Translated by W.G. Spencer. Vol. III Book 8, Loeb Classical library. Harvard University Press. 1938. P 405

Varicose vein surgery.

'Any vein in the leg that is troublesome may be shrivelled by cauterising, or cut by surgery'. To use cautery on moderate sized veins, an incision was made over the vein that was then cauterised with a fine, but blunt hot iron'. This was repeated throughout the length of the vein. If there were large twisted veins, he preferred surgery. This was carried out through incisions four fingers apart down the leg, the vein being retracted with a hook through each incision and cut away.[1] He ligated bleeding veins as necessary.

Reference:

1. *Celsus on Medicine. Vol. III, Book 7.* Loeb Classical library Translated by W.G. Spencer. Harvard University Press. 1938. ISBN 988-0-674-99370-9. P 467.

Excision of impacted urethral stones.

Celsus (c25 BC–c50 AD) describes how to remove a small stone, formed in the bladder that had lodged in the urethra. First, he passed an ear-scoop into the urethra to pull the stone out. If that failed, he then operated by pulling the prepuce over the glans and tying it in place. An incision was made into the urethra and the stone extracted. On releasing the prepuce, the skin returned to its normal position, bringing an intact portion of skin to cover the incision into the urethra and so enabling urine to flow naturally.[1]

Reference:

1. *Celsus on Medicine, Volume II Book VII.* Translated by W.G. Spencer. First published 1938 by Loeb Classical Library. ISBN 988-0-674-99370-9. P 425–427.

First recorded suturing of a laceration of the colon following trauma.

'If the abdomen was penetrated by a stab (wound) and the intestines had then rolled out, it is necessary to see if they are injured and their proper colour persists', wrote Celsus. 'If the smaller intestine has been penetrated (opened), no good could be done'. He then continues. 'The larger intestine can be sutured, not with any certain assurance, but because a doubtful hope is preferable to certain despair, for occasionally it heals up'. Operating on the large bowel electively did not take place until well after the introduction of general anaesthesia in 1846.[1]

Surgery following an abdominal knife wound resulting in the intestines protruding, but undamaged, was described by Abu al-Qasim al-Zahrawi (fl. c1000 AD). The bowel was replaced and the abdominal wall sutured.[2]

References:

1. *Celsus on Medicine. Volume III, Book VII.* Loeb Classical Library, edited by Jeffery Henderson, Harvard University Press 1938. P 385.
2. *Medieval Islamic Medicine.* By Peter E. Pormann & Emily Savage Smith. Edinburgh University Press. 2010. ISBN 988 0 7486 2066 1.

Plastic surgery, reversal of circumcision.

Celsus describes in detail a delicate and ingenious operation to either reverse a circumcision or to form a prepuce in a man in whom it was congenitally absent.

Reference:

1. *Celsus on Medicine. Volume III. Book VII. P* 24. Loeb Classical Library, edited by Jeffery Henderson, Harvard University Press 1938, pp 421 & 423.

Draining of abdominal ascites.

Celsus considered that in, 'Those who are dropsical, the water should be let out'. It was understood that dropsy (ascitic fluid in the abdominal cavity) was generally secondary to a cirrhotic liver. His method to drain it was to make a small incision in the abdomen, four fingers below the umbilicus, taking great care not to inadvertently cut a blood vessel. A bronze tube with a collar round its middle was inserted. The collar was to stop the tube slipping into the abdomen. After releasing some of the ascites, the tube was plugged and bandaged while still remaining in the abdomen so more fluid could be drained daily. The current method for draining ascites is not dissimilar.

Reference:

1. *Celsus on Medicine. Book VII.* Loeb Classical Library, edited by Jeffery Henderson, Harvard University Press 1938, p 383.

Partial thyroidectomy.

Celsus described a 'tumour' in the neck, situated between the skin and the trachea that he called a bronchocele. The Latin translation is 'broncho + cele' or trachea + tumour. Celsus is probably describing a thyroid cyst, which may have degenerated into a honey like liquid. He also records dermoid cysts in the thyroid gland that contained hair and calcified material. Non-surgical treatments were tried first. If these failed then, 'Treatment by the knife is shorter'. A linear incision was made down to the tunic of the thyroid, then the morbid pouch was separated by the finger from the tissue and the whole is removed.[1]

Reference:

Celsus on Medicine. Vol. III, Book 7. Translated by W.G. Spencer. Loeb Classical Library, Harvard University. Edited by Jeffery Henderson, 1938, p 375–377.

Mastectomy.

It is not possible to attribute the first mastectomy to any particular surgeon. Aulus Celsus (c25 BC–c50 AD) mentions cancer of the breast but does not recommend surgery, as he considered it could make the disease worse.[1] This indicates that Celsus was aware of the operation of mastectomy but gives no further information.

A clear description of mastectomy was given by the Greek Byzantine surgeon, Paul of Aegina (625–690) who worked mainly in Arabia in the early years of the Rashidun Caliphate. He describes removal of the breast for cancer, using a knife and cautery. During the Middle Ages, this simple yet dreadful operation persisted, accompanied by cautery or pressure dressings to stem the flow of blood, a technique that was still being practised in 1720 when Lorenz Heister (1683–1758) carried out a similar operation.[2] The use of ligatures to stop vessels bleeding, as advocated by Celus had been forgotten.

During the 18th century, it was recognised by John Hunter (1728-1793) that breast cancer metastasises to the axillary lymph nodes and also less commonly to the lymph nodes of the internal thoracic chain.[3] By 1825, Sir Astley Cooper (1768–1841) recognised that if several of the axillary nodes were involved the disease was then surgically incurable and would inevitably recur. A carefully worded guideline limiting the use of surgery was then produced by Sir James Paget (1814–1899). This cautious approach to operating for cancer of the breast continued until after 1846 when the availability of anaesthesia enabled more radical surgery to be carried out.

In 1882, Dr William Halstead (1852–1922) in the USA was the first to perform a radical mastectomy.[4] He included not only the breast but also the axillary lymph-nodes and pectoralis major muscle in his operation. By the end of the century, he was advocating excision of the supraclavicular nodes although he later abandoned this part of the operation. He produced statistics that 85% of women without lymph-node metastases survived three years, while those with microscopic lymph-node involvement had only a 31% chance of survival.

This radical surgical approach to treatment further increased under Mr W. Samson Handley (1872–1962) of the Middlesex Hospital in London, who hypothesised that cancer spread not only along the lymphatics, but wrongly believed it spread along the tissue planes and so he carried out a very wide excision. This was followed by implanting radium needles along the internal mammary chain. This radical approach lasted until the middle of the 20th century.

Evidence was then gradually accumulating that a simpler operation was as effective. Professor Robert McWhirter (1904–1994) of Edinburgh, compared a large number of patients treated by simple mastectomy followed by radiotherapy, with patients who had undergone radical surgery with radiotherapy. The results were essentially the same.[5] It was also discovered that many metastases were formed by malignant cells that had entered the blood stream and propagated widespread metastases beyond the reach of surgery.

New treatments are now in place consisting of adequate but minimal surgery followed by radiotherapy and chemotherapy.

References:

1. *Celsus on Medicine. Vol. 111.* Translated by W.G. Spencer. Loeb Classical Library. Harvard University Press, 1938. P 592.
2. *A History of Surgery.* By Harold Ellis. 2001. Greenwich Medical Media Ltd. London. ISBN. 1-84110-023-4.
3. *Hunterian Reminiscences, being the substance of a course of Lectures on the Principles and Practice of Surgery delivered by John Hunter in the Year 1785.* By James Parkinson. Edited by P. W. K. Parkinson in 1888. Nabu Public Domain Books. P.158–161.
4. *Genius on the Edge. The bizarre double life of Dr William Stewart Halstead.* By Gerald Imber MD. Kaplan Publishing, New York. 2011. P 121–126.

5. No Ordinary Meeting: Robert McWhirter and the decline of radical mastectomy. J R Coll Physicians Edinb. Newmark J.J., 2016 Mar; 46(1): 43–48.

Excision of hydrocele

A hydrocele is a collection of fluid in that part of the peritoneum that descended with the testis into the scrotum. When permanent large and tense, Celsus advised surgery.

Reference:

Celsus on Medicine. Vol. III. Translated by W.G. Spencer. Loeb Classical Library. Harvard University Press, Cambridge, Massachusetts, USA. 1938. p 395–407.

c79 AD. Rome. The first hospitals.

In the first century AD, the Roman Empire expanded considerably and the distance to its frontiers correspondingly increased. Military commanders needed to provide special quarters dedicated to the care and treatment of the sick and wounded. These were the first hospitals. They were known as 'valetudinaria'[1] and 25 have been excavated along the frontiers of the Roman Empire from Scotland to Palestine. All were built to a standard plan.

They were constructed around a quadrangle with a corridor on the inside. In an archaeological excavation of the ancient Roman military camp in Inchtuthil in central Scotland, it was discovered that this valetudinarium had sixty-four rooms or wards, each accommodating four to five men, so the hospital could accommodate 220 sick or wounded soldiers. Greek military surgeons mainly staffed the medical corps.[2] When the Western Roman Empire was finally overrun, the valetudinaria fell into decay and were forgotten.

The instruments used by the surgeons serving these hospitals would have been similar to those discovered during excavations of Pompeii, destroyed in the volcanic eruption of Vesuvius in 79 AD. They included scalpels, forceps, tissue hooks, a male catheter of bronze, saws and specula with a screw ratchet, similar to those used in modern gynaecological examinations. There were delicate probes,[3] but there was no evidence of a hospital in either Pompeii or Herculaneum.

An earlier claim to have the earliest hospital has been made for King Ashoka (c261 BC) of the Maurya Dynasty in India whose edict carved in stone is thought to have referred to a hospital. Dr Guido Majno finds this claim rests on a single word, 'chikisaka', which has been interpreted by one translator as a hospital, but other translators describe it as referring only to 'remedies'.[4]

In the early Christian era, hospitals called 'xenodochia' were built. The most famous was founded by St Basil in Caesarea in Cappadocia in 372 AD. It was custom built and designed for its purpose with space for expansion.

The first public hospital founded in the West was in about 390 AD and was situated at Ostia, Rome's port. It became famous and excavations in the 20th century rediscovered the hospital's foundations that measured 58 metres in length.[5]

A major hospital was built in the 9th century in Iraq by the Arab Nestorian Patriarch, Timothy 1 (d. 823). It was situated in the southeast of Baghdad and was very grand. In 982, the Adudi hospital was established and staffed by 25 doctors. It was later described as having many 'chambers and rooms and all the appurtenances of a royal residence'. The Caliph al-Muqtadir (r. 908–932) established more hospitals in Baghdad in the 910s and 920s. Hospitals were also built in Granada in Muslim Spain in 1399.[6] The medical needs of the wealthy continued to be provided in their private houses which probably explains why relatively few hospitals seem to have been built.

References:

1. *The Healing Hand.* By Guido Majno. Harvard University Press 1985. P. 385.
2. Ibid., P 390.
3. Wikipedia. Excavation of Pompeii.
4. *The Healing Hand.* By Guido Majno. Harvard University Press 1985. P. 264–265.
5. *Science Medicine and History. Essays on the Evolution of Scientific Thought and Medical Practice.* Written in honour of Charles Singer. Volume One edited by E. Ashworth Underwood. Book I. The Origin of Hospitals by George E Gask and John Todd. Oxford University Press, 1953. P. 129.

6. *Medieval Islamic Medicine.* By P.E. Pormann and Emilie Savage-Smith. Edinburgh University Press, 2007, ISBN 988 0 7486 2066 1.

c120 AD. Rome. Soranus of. The first vaginal hysterectomy.

Soranus of Ephesus is known to have been active in about 120 AD and is believed to have died before Galen wrote his *De Methoda Medendi* which has been dated to approximately 178 AD. Soranus wrote a treatise on *Gynaecology and Paediatrics* and was the foremost physician of his time. Like most surgeons in the Roman Empire, he was a Greek and practiced in Rome.[1]

He wrote extensively concerning non-surgical treatment of a prolapsed uterus. He also advocated surgery 'when the uterus is permanently prolapsed' and 'if part of the uterus has turned black…one should cut off the black part. If the whole uterus has become black, one must cut it off in its entirety', so giving the first description of a vaginal hysterectomy.

The first abdominal hysterectomy took place in 1853, early in the post anaesthetic era.[2]

References:

1. *Soranus' Gynecology.* Translated by Owsei Temkin. Published by Johns Hopkins Press, Baltimore, US. Paperback edition 1991, p 207.
2. Abdominal Hysterectomy. Ch. 2. Index and Timeline. 1853.

c. 150 AD. Antyllus. Brachial artery aneurysm ligation.

Little is known of Antyllus[1] (f c150 AD) except that he lived in the same era as Galen. Where Galen excelled in anatomy, physiology and medicine. Antyllus' was the first to describe the operations for aneurysms and tracheostomy. His surgical expertise has come to us from Oribasius (320–403) a Byzantine surgeon who copied these operations.

The successor surgeon who gives a good description of aneurysm surgery was Aetius of Amida (502-572) who was physician to Justinian 1 (482-575) the Roman Emperor of Byzantium. Aetius describes an aneurysm at the elbow and instructs that the artery feeding it is tied a hands breath below the armpit. The aneurysm is then exposed, opened and the blood clot evacuated, then the artery immediately above and below the aneurysm was tied.

The instructions are clear and could be followed by another surgeon of that time provided he had appropriate anatomical knowledge. Suppuration of all wounds was expected and accepted as normal. Aetius calls it 'good suppuration', it was later called 'laudable pus' until the 20th century.[2]

Antyllus' operation must be compared with that of John Hunter (1728–1793), who in December 1785 performed the same operation on an aneurysm behind the knee, by tying the artery above the aneurysm leaving the collateral circulation to 'nourish' the parts below the ligature. Hunter was well versed in experiments on animals and it is just possible he independently came to the same conclusion as Antyllus of his own accord[3]

This is possible but still leaves Antyllus as having been the first to carry out this original operation. Sir Stephen Paget in 1847 considered Hunter's operation to be an original operation, but it was not claimed as such by Hunter himself. It appears that Paget was unaware of Antyllus or that Aetius 1200 years earlier, had also carried out this operation.

References:

1. *History of Medicine, Vol. 1.* By Max Neuburger translated by Ernest Playfair. London, Henry Frowde, OUP. 1910. Reprinted by Forgotten Books. App Store, p 274.
2. *A History of Surgery*. By Harold Ellis, 2001. Greenwich Medical Media Ltd. ISBN 1-84110-023-4.*3. Masters of Medicine: John Hunter, Man of Science and Surgeon.* By Stephen Paget, Sir James Paget and Ernest Hart. Leopold Classic library, originally printed in 1847.

c. 150 AD. Antyllus. First tracheostomy

Antyllus was the first to carry out a tracheostomy.[1] As in the previous entry, this operation was attributed to him by Orobasius (320–403) who also carried out this operation.

Paul of Aegina (c625–c690) was a Greek who wrote a *Medical Compendium* in seven books, possibly while in Alexandria before the Muslim conquest. He was later given an Arabic name, Al-kawabeli, the Accoucheur. His texts in Greek were later translated into Arabic by Hunayn Ibn Ishaq al-Ibadi(809–873). Paul was the last of the Greek surgeons to write about tracheostomies.

From a modern surgical point of view, it may be surmised that on seeing the patient he had immediately proceeded to carry out the tracheostomy as it was an obvious emergency. He bent the head backwards, to make the trachea more accessible. He then made an incision and cut between the third and fourth rings of the trachea. This saved the man's life.

One helpful fact given is that on opening the trachea there was a hissing noise as air rushed into the lungs. For this to happen, the patient must have exhausted the oxygen in his lungs and become cyanosed, gone a deep blue colour. There was no time to operate on the tonsils which were obstructing his airway as the man was about to die. The tonsils must have been obstructing the airway, so he must have followed the tracheostomy by a tonsillectomy, as he was able to close the tracheostomy.[2]

Another account of tracheostomy was by Ibn Zuhr(d. 1162) who practised in Muslim Spain. He describes a tracheostomy on a goat and wrote that as he had never seen the operation carried out on a human.[3]

There have been suggestions that a tracheostomy was performed in pre-dynastic ancient Egypt (31st century BC). The description of the suggested operation cannot be anatomically reconciled with a tracheostomy operation and may have represented human sacrifice.[4] Surgery at that time was simple and primitive and as such a tracheostomy at that date can be dismissed.

Tracheostomies are now commonplace in patients needing prolonged ventilation in Intensive Care Units.

References:

1. *History of Medicine, Vol. 1.* By Max Neuburger translated by Ernest Playfair. London, Henry Frowde, OUP. 1910. Reprinted by Forgotten Books. App Store, p 274
2. *The End of the Golden Age of general Surgery. 1870–2000.* By N.K. Maybury. Printed by Amazon 2014. ISBN 13: 9781499531374, p 37.
3. *Medieval Islamic Medicine.* By Peter E. Pormann & Emily Savage Smith. Edinburgh University Press. 2010. ISBN 978 0 7486 2066 1.
4. Bloomstedt, P. Tracheostomy in ancient Egypt. J. Laryngol. Otol. Aug; 128(8): 665–8. 2014.

c180 AD. Rome. Claudius Galen of Pergamon and the transmission of his work.

Galen (130–c200 AD) was a Roman of Greek origin from the Roman Province of Asia Minor. While his medicine was essentially Hippocratic (c460–c377 BC), his surgery was more sophisticated than that of Hippocrates in that he was a successor surgeon who improved many of Hippocrates' original operations.

Galen's education is interesting because he became the most famous anatomist and surgeon of his time and influenced the practice of surgery for the next 1500 years. His father wanted to prepare him for a career in the service of Rome, but he had a dream that turned his attention to medicine. Having listened to, and wearied of, philosophers setting out different and conflicting views, he shifted his attention to mathematics and then anatomy. While in his teens, he studied in Pergamon for four years under Satyros, an anatomist of that time. He then went to Smyrna to pursue his anatomical studies and wrote a treatise in three books on the thorax and lungs. Following this, he travelled to Alexandria in Egypt, the most important scientific centre of the Roman Empire. In Alexandria, he carried out the first accurately recorded physiological experiments. In 158 following twelve years of medical studies, he returned to Pergamon and was appointed surgeon to the gladiators.[1]

Galen spoke Greek throughout his life and was born in the golden age of the Roman Empire where Greek was the language of philosophy and medicine, while Latin was the language of administration, commerce and the military. The educated classes often spoke both languages. Galen's written output ran to about two million words. These were preserved and studied by Byzantine physicians and were translated into Syriac and then Arabic. His work on medicine and surgery became the basis of Arabic medicine in the Caliphates of both East and West[2] and later were translated into Latin and transmitted to Italy, and soon afterwards into Western Europe.

References:

1. *Galen of Pergamon* By George Sarton. University of Kansas Press 1954. Library of Congress number: 54–8112.
2. *Galen on the Natural Faculties.* By Arthur John Brock, 2016, Erik Publications.

On the suture of muscles and tendons.

This is Galen's (130–c200 AD) only original operation. He returned to Pergamon in 158 as physician and surgeon to the gladiators.[1] There, he recorded his observations of the trauma inflicted on them. Celsus (c25 BC–c50 AD), had previously observed severed or disrupted tendons were common in the arena, but Galen was the first to suture and reconnect these tissues. It was believed at that time that tendons contracted and due to their similar appearance, they could be confused with nerves with unfortunate results. The action of muscles was not then understood.[2] Galen followed Celsus' lead by ligating bleeding arteries in wounded gladiators and thereby reduced the number of fatalities.

References:

1. *Galen of Pergamon* By George Sarton. University of Kansas Press 1954. Library of Congress Catalogue Card Number 54–8112.
2. *Galen on the Usefulness of Parts of the Body.* Translated by M.T. May, Cornell University press 1968. 2 vols.

Anatomical advances

Galen would have known that Aristotle (384–322 BC) had dissected over a hundred species of animals as described in *Historia Animalium.*[1] In Galen's time, it was forbidden to dissect human bodies and like Aristotle, he dissected animals. His dissections were meticulous and the most accurate to that date.

His detailed anatomical studies, especially of the Barbary ape 'Macaca inius', were carried out due to their similarity to man.[2] Unsurprisingly, there were significant anatomical differences between humans and the apes that caused problems in later ages when Galen's anatomy was used as the standard textbook of anatomy for surgeons. The most troublesome differences were of the skull and the female pelvis. The latter causing puzzlement and probably despair among midwives, as they tried to align the human and ape pelvis when attending women at childbirth. Galen's detailed anatomical knowledge did enable him to accurately perform physiological experiments.

References:

1. *The Works of Aristotle Translated into English. Historia Animalia.* By D'Arcy Wentworth Thompson. Oxford at the Clarendon Press 1910.
2. *Galen on Anatomical Procedures.* Translation of the Surviving Books by Charles Singer. Oxford University Press 1956, Special Edition for Sandpiper Books Ltd., 1999.

The first physiological experiments. Galen (129 or 130–c200 AD) carried out carefully planned physiological experiments. These included opening arteries in live animals, that proved for the first time that they only contained blood, and not blood and air as had been previously thought when arteries had been opened post-mortem. Galen did not understand the function of the heart and believed that blood was formed in the liver and flowed into the veins.

In experiments on a live pig, he ligated the ureters to demonstrate that they fill with urine, proving for the first time that urine originates in the kidneys, a fact previously disputed.[1] Separately, he tied an animal's urethra, to demonstrate that when the bladder was full and distended the ureters did not also distend due to backflow from the bladder. The mechanism preventing backflow was discovered centuries later when it was recognised that the ureters pass through the bladder wall obliquely. Then, when the bladder fills and distends with urine, the bladder muscles stretch and compress the lower end of the ureters, effectively closing them and preventing back flow, while allowing urine to pass into the bladder. This was the first demonstration of a 'flutter valve'.

In another entirely original series of experiments, he discovered and proved that the brain controls all the activity of the muscles through the cranial and peripheral nervous systems. To demonstrate this, Galen severed in sequence different nerves or portions of the spinal cord at different levels of a pig's vertebral column. He observed and described the exact extent and distribution of the subsequent paralysis that each incision caused.[2] In one such experiment, he severed the recurrent laryngeal nerves noting that 'with the nerves damaged, the animal becomes dumb'.[3] His experiments significantly advanced the knowledge of anatomy and physiology through his studies of structure and function. These experiments were cruel. In mitigation, surgeons before the discovery of anaesthesia one-thousand six-hundred years later, had to be composed and unruffled while they operated on patients who were suffering agonising pain and who had to be held down throughout an operation.

Also, as surgeon to the gladiators in Pergamum for several years he must have been hardened to the cruelty of man. It is reputed that his skill as their surgeon significantly reduced the mortality from wounds inflicted in the arena. After his lengthy training, experimentation and extensive travel Galen settled in Rome, spending five years as a military surgeon and was later appointed physician to Commodus,[4] the son of the Roman Emperor Marcus Aurelius (121–180) after whose death, he continued to attend Commodus as Emperor.

References:

1. *The Healing Hand.* By Guido Majno. Harvard University Press, 1975.
2. *Galen on the Usefulness of Parts of the Body.* Translated by M.T. May, Cornell University Press 1968. 2 vols.
3. *Galen on Anatomical Procedures* Translation of the Surviving Books by Charles Singer. Oxford University Press 1956. ISBN: 0-19-924016-7.
4. *Galen of Pergamon* By George Sarton. University of Kansas Press. 1954, p 23.

Galen observed that a few wounds healed without sepsis.

Galen[1] (130–c200 AD) was the greatest surgeon of his age. It was in Pergamon that he treated wounded gladiators by suturing severed tendons and muscles and ligating bleeding blood vessels. He also noted and recorded that a few wounds healed by 'first intention', that is without sepsis[1] the aim of all modern surgeons.

Galen's interesting observation that wounds could heal without sepsis was lost to posterity. In the Ancient Greek language, the same word means both wound and ulcer, the latter is by definition an infected wound.[2] Not surprising, nearly all wounds until Lister's time became septic and this was accepted as normal. Even in the nineteenth century, physicians were still talking about 'laudable pus'.

References:

1. *Galen of Pergamon* By George Sarton. University of Kansas Press 1954. Library of Congress Catalogue Card Number 54–8112.
2. *The Healing Hand.* By Guido Majno. Harvard University Press, 1975, p 400.

410 AD. The fall of Rome and the beginning of the Dark Ages in the West.

When Alaric the Goth sacked Rome in 410, the Western Roman Empire was already in steep decline and with its fall, the art of surgery in the West came to an end. What had been learned by the Greeks and Romano-Greeks was now forgotten. For example, the practice of tying bleeding arteries was lost. There was no training and dissection was forbidden on religious grounds and disease was once again thought to be the result of sin causing divine displeasure.[1]

In Anglo-Saxon England, between the 5th and the middle of the 11th century the duty of care to the sick was managed by the Church. The main source of information concerning this period came from the Venerable Bede, a monk in Durham in the North East of England. The Church possessed copies of some Ancient Greek authors, but we do not know which ones or that they were studied, as they were later destroyed in Viking attacks.

Disease during those times, according to the Church, was a punishment for sin. After the sinner had repented came forgiveness, it was then the Church's duty to remove and cure the disease. Cutting with the knife is mentioned but no specific operation is described except venesection.[2] Cautery was used, but for what ailment we do not know. This illustrates that Anglo-Saxon surgery was virtually non-existent.

Meanwhile, the study of medicine and surgery was beginning in Salerno in southern Italy. A classic age of scholarship followed the arrival of a Carthaginian scholar, Constantine the African, who translated the Arabic renditions of Hippocrates and Galen's works into Latin[3] for the first time beginning in 1077.

References:

1. *A History of Surgery.* By Harold Ellis, 2001. Greenwich Medical Media Ltd. ISBN 1-84110-023-4.

2. *General Medical Practice in Anglo-Saxon England.* By Wilfred Bonsor. Science and History of Medicine. Essays on the evolution of thought and medical practice. Volume One. Edited by E. Ashworth Underwood. Oxford University Press. 1953.
3. Wikipedia. Constantine Africanus.

Chapter 6

Greek Philosophy of Medicine and Surgery

The overwhelming and enduring influence of Greek thought on medicine and surgery that reached Western Europe in the Middle Ages was practised into the early modern period. Even today, the echoes of their knowledge can be found buried in the background of modern surgery when operations are undertaken on the superficial tissues of the body. Over the last few centuries, their principles and approach to surgery have been examined in detail by learned English and continental scholars. The importance of the subject to surgery is unquestionable and what follows is a summary and explanation of their conclusions.

Their theories began when the Ancient Greek philosophers laid down the rules for structured argument and disputation. This established a complete break with the past, that enabled them to discuss ideas rationally for the first time.[1] These ideas were forged in the freedom of the Greek City States beginning in Miletus in Asia Minor, where belief in the omniscience of the gods to control the daily lives of people was for the first time rejected.

As their ideas developed, the Ancient Greeks thought that medical doctrines were also philosophic in nature, since the actual causes of disease were unknown and remained so into the middle of the 19th century. Paradoxically, the Greeks began to believe that what they thought was actually fact. Only because they had 'visualised it in their mind's eye' or through 'the sight of the mind'[2]

Logic was then a new intellectual tool and initially poorly understood, for it resulted in hypotheses often being treated as facts.[3] They considered that thought was the physical exercise of the soul, that could temporarily leave the body and 'walk abroad'. It was as though they were trying to explain nature by 'shutting their eyes', confirming it as purely an exercise for the intellect. Through these mental exercises, they gradually produced a theoretical explanation for the origin of diseases, as well as a framework within which to practice both medicine and surgery. One example being that it explained why wounds produced 'laudable' pus.[4]

This process started when Thales[5] of Miletus (662–546 BC), the founder of the first Greek school of philosophy, asked himself of what the world and everything in it was made. His answer was both ingenious and wrong. He opted for 'water' as the prime constituent of the world. After all, it is to be found everywhere, falling from the sky, disgorged by streams and rivers into the sea, frozen on mountains and when heated it becomes a gas. Furthermore, water is essential for all life. Thales came to this conclusion through his 'mind's eye' and it became the first of the new ideas proposed by the Ancient Greeks.

Thales' abstract reasoning was a constant feature of Greek thought and with it the belief that the physical and moral universe must be simple, rational and therefore knowable. He believed that the apparent multiplicity of physical things in the world were only superficial and could be broken down into earth, fire, air and water from which everything in the world was made.

Then, Anaximander of Miletus[6] (c610–c546 BC) produced another philosophical idea. He described the concept of an 'unidentified something' which had no substance, but contained 'opposites' within itself such as, hot and cold, and wet and dry. His theory was predicated on the idea that normality, including health, was a balance between opposites in nature. Too much or too little, of either hot or cold, or of wet or dry or any combination of them, caused an imbalance in the body's constitution. This led to disequilibrium that showed itself as a disease. This was the theory of the 'four humours' and was accepted by Hippocrates over a century later, who then associated it with the four elements.

Another ancient concept was the idea of a soul. Pythagoras[7] (c570–c495 BC) thought the soul was divided into three parts, consciousness, the mind or reason and emotion. The first and last he considered common to all animals and the second to man alone. Although initially thought to be in the heart, the mind came to be considered as the seat of the soul or 'life force' and was centred in the brain, along with consciousness and the bodily senses. The emotions remained in the heart. He believed that reason and the mind were the same thing and were eternal, while the body was mortal. Speculation also led Pythagoras to believe that air was equated with the soul. He reasoned that the soul was nourished by the blood and it was blood that connects the whole body via the arteries and veins. The trachea at that time was included with the blood vessels, as it was believed to deliver air to the heart by means of some passage that was then believed existed. Pythagoras complicated things by postulating that the air was full of spirits, good and bad that sent men their dreams and diseases. [8]Heraclitus (c540–c480 BC) in about 500 BC produced a counter-intuitive thought. He stated that since we cannot absolutely trust our senses, we can never really trust them at all.[9] His idea was that things that appear solid are actually undergoing gradual and constant change into something else. He believed everything was in ceaseless flux. Obviously, he knew that wood rots and living creatures die and decompose. Such observations led to his idea that all matter was in a state of constant flux. His belief in the limitations of human sense organs has been confirmed by modern science, with the discovery that human vision is limited to only a small part of the total spectrum between ultra-violet and infra-red.

A little later, Alcmaeon of Croton (f c450 BC) discovered the optic nerve, leading him to associate sight with the brain, that strengthened the view that the brain was the seat of consciousness. He apparently came to this conclusion when attending a patient with a severe injury resulting in the extrusion of an eyeball that he amputated revealing its anatomical attachment.

He also taught that disease was caused by disequilibrium of the normally balanced qualities of the constitution. He argued that humans were the only example of rational beings and agreed that the brain was the seat of the mind and intelligence. While he still believed the heart was the seat of the soul and the genital organs were the origin of them all. Because he said 'they all sprout and grow from them'.[9] His difference from Pythagoras over the location of the soul was settled in favour of the brain being the seat of intelligence two centuries later at Alexandria in Egypt.

From his dissections, Alcmaeon had recognised that there was a distinction between the function of the arteries and the veins. He observed that the principal arteries contained very little blood after death. He was unaware that after death most of the arterial blood flowed into the venous system due to its initial muscular contraction. So, when he opened arteries post-mortem, they appeared to have only a few blood clots and air in them. From this, he wrongly concluded that in a living animal the arteries carried pneuma or air that was directly breathed into the blood through the brain by way of supposed pores in the nose, by which it entered the arteries.[10]

The veins meanwhile were believed to carry nutrition in the blood to and from the liver. This strange dichotomy, associated with a lack of understanding of the anatomy of the distribution of the arteries that enter every organ and the veins that leave every organ, was a major factor in delaying the discovery of the circulation of the blood. [11]

Empedocles of Acragas(f. 445 BC) is believed to have anticipated Aristotle in his discovery that the heart, and not the brain, is the first organ to develop in an embryo. He observed a chick embryo during the third and fourth days of its development and saw movement of the heart and vessels with the naked eye. That the heart was the first organ to develop was of special interest and made him identify it with the 'soul' that he considered eternal. [12] He carried out his most prolific work in Alexandria

in Egypt and influenced science for many centuries. He supported the theory of the four elements of water, earth, air and fire and the four humours of hot and cold and wet and dry. He declared all these could be identified through the sense of touch. An idea later accepted by Hippocrates. This is now supported by recent discoveries from the Cambrian Era that show the sense of touch was the earliest of the sense organs to evolve in animal life half a billion years ago. [13]

Hippocrates (460–370 BC) then formulated and formalised the Greek theory of disease that took place when the elements were no longer balanced in health but had fallen into a state of disequilibrium. He considered that in practical terms this could cause a flux or movement of fluid from one tissue to another in the body.

He wrote that 'Fluxes occur when the tissues of the body become over-chilled or over heated'. In either case, a disease is developed due to an imbalance between any of the hot and cold or wet and dry elements. 'A flux that arises from excessive cold brings on shivering (and) contraction of the tissues that squeezes out its moisture'. He used as an example of a flux, the nasal discharge during a common cold. Fluxes also arose from excessive heat and he conjectured that tissues on becoming hot develop passages within them, through which the heated moisture then flows in the direction of least resistance. Hippocrates gave the knee joint as an example. [14] 'For when moisture flows out of the tissues and into a joint that does not have room for it, the cords (ligaments) being stretched, unbinds the joint, making the person lame'. Another example was an 'excess of phlegm and of dryness brings on a flux'. In the latter case, it draws excess moisture to the area of dryness.

From this, it can be gathered that fluxes follow an imbalance in any of the classic elements, wet/dry, hot/cold, and can also be interpreted as an imbalance of blood and phlegm, or yellow and black bile. With this theory, any pain, lump, fever or wound could be considered a disharmony and therefore a disease. This was Hippocrates' unifying theory of disease and is generally known as the theory of the four humours.

Of course, the Hippocratic idea of a disease, as described above was only a hypothesis. Hippocrates first used the word 'hypothesis' in his treatise *On Ancient Medicine,* when the concept was in its infancy. [15] His hypothesis on the nature of disease soon came to be treated as 'fact' and was accepted as such into the late medieval period. Hippocrates' ideas were only displaced by the discoveries of the actual causes of disease in the 19th and 20th centuries.

Be that as it may, to appreciate the advance made by Hippocrates when he declared that disease was a 'natural phenomenon' was a fundamental break from all that had gone before. His achievement of separating disease from the magic of Egypt, or the view that health and disease were in the hands of the gods and therefore inexplicable was a significant advance. This also applies to the advances made by the Ancient Greek philosophers already mentioned.

For to understand the scale of all these achievements, they must be compared with earlier beliefs and not with modern science or medicine. For Hippocrates' achievements propelled the School of Medicine on the Island of Cos, along with his written documents on medicine and surgery to the forefront of knowledge at that time.

To this was added his insistence that those taking his 'Oath' before practising medicine must act with probity and in the best interests of their patients. This contributed to his being called the Father of Medicine. Hippocrates' treatises survived due to the interest taken in them by successive civilisations in the total absence of more plausible ideas. This was why his ideas remained the principal theory of disease for nearly 2300 years, that is until pus was discovered to be of pathogenic bacterial origin.

We now digress to consider Aristotle of Stagira (384–322 BC), the founder of 'natural science'. When seventeen, he had been sent by his father to study under Plato at the Academy in Athens and stayed for twenty years until Plato's death in 347 BC. He then travelled and spent time on the Island of Lesbos where he studied a wide variety of creatures from the sea, land and air. This familiarised him with their forms, similarities and differences, both through observation and dissection. His treatise, *Historia Animalium*, is an extraordinary book, as none like it had ever been written before. He broke the mould of pure philosophy with his systematic observation of nature. He appreciated and understood the similarities as well as the differences in the animal world. It was he who was the first to describe species and recognise the similarity of some animals, later to be grouped together and designated as genera. [16]

Like Empedocles, nearly a century earlier, he studied the development of a chick embryo. He also observed that the heart was the first organ to develop, but unlike Empedocles who identified the blood with the soul Aristotle concluded that the heart was both the seat of intelligence and as it was the first organ to develop was also the seat of the soul. On observing the perpetual pulsation of the heart and arteries, while knowing nothing about capillaries invisible to the naked eye, he agreed with the existing theory that the blood moved up and down the blood vessels. Aristotle like Empedocles was also searching for the life force that is transmitted between generations.[17]

Aristotle accepted that when the elements, hot and cold and wet and dry, are in equilibrium, then good health results, while imbalance of these leads to disease. He thought that sleep was due to the moderate cooling of the blood and that complete absence of heat in the blood resulted in death.

The foregoing description of the development of Ancient Greek philosophy led to a theory that was a purely intellectual concept. The next chapter describes the practicalities of its practice and its drawbacks, including the liberal use of venesection.

References:

1. *Ancient Culture and Society. Early Greek Science: Thales to Aristotle.* By G.E.R. Lloyd. Chatto and Windus, 1982. London. p 1-2.
2. *The Healing Hand: Man and Wound in the Ancient world.* By Guido Majno, MD. Harvard University Press. 1975. P. 181.
3. *Hippocrates on Ancient Medicine.* Translated by Francis Adams. Printed in GB by Amazon. ISBN 978-153572558. P. 5.
4. *The Healing Hand: Man and Wound in the Ancient world.* By Guido Majno, MD. Harvard University Press. 1975. P. 102.
5. *The Greeks.* By H.D.F. Kitto. Penguin Books, Harmondsworth, Middlesex. Reprinted 1954. p 178.

6. *Ancient Culture and Society. Early Greek Science: Thales to Aristotle.* By G.E.R. Lloyd. Chatto and Windus, London. 1982. Anaximander of Miletus (610-546 BCE) p. 20.
7. *The Heart and Vascular System in Ancient Greek Medicine, From Alcmaeon to Galen.* By C.R.S. Harris. Oxford at the Clarendon Press. 1983. Pythagorus. p. 9-10.
8. *The Heart and Vascular System in Ancient Greek Medicine, From Alcmaeon to Galen.* By C.R.S. Harris. Oxford at the Clarendon Press. 1983. P. 10-11.
9. *The Heart and Vascular System in Ancient Greek Medicine,* by C.R.S. Harris. Oxford at the Clarendon Press. ISBN 0-19-858135-1. 1983. P. 6.
10. *The Heart and Vascular System in Ancient Greek Medicine,* by C.R.S. Harris. Oxford at the Clarendon Press. ISBN 0-19-858135-1. 1983. 7-8.
11. *The Heart and Vascular System in Ancient Greek Medicine,* by C.R.S. Harris. Oxford at the Clarendon Press. ISBN 0-19-858135-1. 1983. P. 8.
12. *The Heart and Vascular System in Ancient Greek Medicine,* by C.R.S. Harris. Oxford at the Clarendon Press. ISBN 0-19-858135-1. 1983.The immortality of the soul. P. 11.
13. *The Ancient Origins of Consciousness*, How the brain created experience, by Feinberg T.E. and Mallett J.M. The MIT Press, Cambridge, Massachusetts. 2017. ISBN. 9880262034333. P. 30, 40.
14. *Hippocrates. Volume V111.* Editor and Translator, Paul Potter. Loeb Classical Library. Harvard University Press. 1995, Places in Man, Joints. p. 35-39.
15. *Hippocrates. On Ancient Medicine.* Translated by Francis Adams. ISBN 13: 978-1535372558. P. 13-14.
16. The Works of Aristotle translated into English. Vol. IV *Historia Animalium.* Translated by D'Arcy Wentworth Thompson. Published, Oxford at the Clarendon Press. 1910.
17. *The Beginning of Western Science. The European Scientific Tradition. 600 BC to AD 1450.* By David C Lindberg. University of Chicago Press. 1992. P 64-65.

Chapter 7

Ancient Egyptian and Greek Theories of Disease and Treatment

Bleeding patients by venesection as a treatment was Greek in origin, but the theory that supported its use started in Ancient Egypt in or before 1,700 BC. The Egyptian theory was that following a wound or injury, 'bad blood' collected around a wound and was a major cause of disease. This is an earlier example of a flux already described by Hippocrates.

The Egyptians also believed that, once food had been digested, the residue in the colon and rectum contained putrid substances that were another cause of disease. Their knowledge of anatomy was rudimentary, for they thought that blood vessels were collected together in two parts of the body. The first was around the heart and the second was wrongly believed to be around the rectum. They believed that an imagined rectal network of blood vessels absorbed faecal material that went on to cause disease. Once these 'poisons' had entered and mixed with the blood, they decayed together and penetrated the flesh, which was when the disease became apparent.[1] To try to avoid these diseases, that might now be thought of as the first example of prophylactic medicine, a dedicated specialist physician who was called 'the Shepherd of the Anus',[2] had many recipes for enemas with which to keep the rectum clean. It was customary for important people to have their bowels purged three times a month according to Herodotus.

1. The ancient Greek theory of disease and treatment by venesection.

Hippocrates (460–370 BC), while not accepting the rectum as a source of disease, accepted the Ancient Egyptian idea that blood when mixed with a noxious agent leaves the blood vessels and penetrates the surrounding flesh to decay and become the disease itself. It also involved the theory of the four humours.[3] When a person was in a state of health, the humours were balanced in equilibrium. However, when a wound, injury, fever or other severe adverse condition took place the intrinsic humours became unbalanced, resulting in a state of disequilibrium or disease. These pathways producing disease always resulted in the same treatment being administered.

The first of Hippocrates' pathways was when blood stagnated in the flesh, either around a wound or close to it. He thought that this blood, after leaving the arteries near the wound, caused the tissues to swell. As it decayed, it turned into 'bad blood', that was the disease itself. The treatment was to drain it, which Hippocrates thought was best accomplished by venesection.[4]

The second pathway for disease to occur was also in the 'flesh' that consisted of fat, muscles, nerves and tendons. Although at that time, these tissues were undifferentiated and thought to be single mass. The disease irritating this flesh could cause spasms or convulsions, precipitated by either extreme cold or possibly excessive purging. Purging often followed the administration of a dose of Hellebore to clear a patient's bowels. Hellebore, a poisonous plant, was frequently used until modern times as a medicine, even though an overdose could produce convulsions or death, complications difficult to avoid, for it was not then possible to accurately calibrate doses of medicines. These convulsions and spasms in the flesh attracted blood from the arteries that then 'decayed'. An idea that led to the practice of keeping wounds warm to avoid the development of spasms or convulsions and so discourage blood from being attracted out of the blood vessels, in the hope it would reduce the likelihood of decay and disease.[5]

From this came the Greek's mistaken belief that the swelling around a wound was caused by bad blood. Modern pathology teaches us that following an injury white cells accompanied by serum pass through the walls of the capillaries to make their way to destroy pathogenic bacteria and this causes the swelling, a fact completely unknown until after 1858 when the germ theory of disease was proved.

His mind free and untainted by the discoveries of the future, Hippocrates followed the theory of disease caused by disequilibrium of the humours. They filled the void he had created when he had rejected the belief that the gods were the source of diseases inflicted on humans as punishment. He correctly thought that disease was a natural phenomenon and in the context of his times, the theory of the humours was a satisfactory categorisation.

By understanding this, the reader might just for a moment, be persuaded to accept Hippocrates' theory that disease was caused by decayed and stagnating blood. If this can be accepted, as it has been by untold thousands of physicians, surgeons and patients in the past, then it was not totally illogical to open a vein nearby to drain the bad blood. This was reinforced by the belief that blood travelled separately up and down the arteries and veins. This was the rationale for performing venesection and fits with Hippocrates theory that 'the wound is the disease'.[6]

The theoretical elegance of Hippocrates' causes of disease, resulted in venesection being the single treatment applicable to any supposed disequilibrium of the humours. It could be applied to an injury, chest infection, abdominal pain, fever or any other disease. To treat all these imbalances, venesection came to be believed as the cure. It could have a calming effect on the patient who may have been grateful that something was being done to help them, for the placebo effect cannot be dismissed.

To perform venesection, Hippocrates laid down the rules. 'Bleed the patient to get rid of bad humours, starve the patient to prevent further bad humours and finally purge the patient to get rid of any other ill humours as might infest the bowel'. Dr Guido Majno[7] in his book published in 1975 asked why was it that, 'Nobody worried that the good humours might go out with the bad'?

There was of course no truth in the Greek theory of humours. Generally, it can be agreed that 'Greek medicine, great as it was as an art, was a failure as a science'. Greek physicians studied disease primarily by giving it a lot of thought, and as has already been noted were accused of trying to explain nature with their eyes shut.[8] Despite this, the theory of humours stood as a framework within which a physician or surgeon could practice and use venesection as the treatment for virtually any illness. It was a malign treatment that never cured anyone, but its use continued into the 20th century. During 2300 years, its frequent and often repeated use on ill patients weakened them further and must have sent untold numbers to an early grave.

However, the fact that the majority of patients survived this 'treatment' was taken as proof of its success. This was of course wrong and it is perhaps ironic and fitting to note that in Greece, the homeland of venesection, Lord George Gordon Byron (1788–1824) who passionately campaigned to liberate the Greeks from the Turks, died in Greece following venesection to 'treat' a fever'!

The rules for venesection as laid down by Hippocrates clearly stated that, 'The cuts (into the vein) should be as close as possible to the determined source of pain,' or disease. His examples included the practice that venesection for pains in the side were to be relieved by an incision into a vein in the hollow of the knee or at the ankle on the same side of the body. For a patient with pain in the right side of the chest venesection was to take place at the elbow on the same side. In addition, emetics and purging that were also malign treatments, continued as staples of ancient medicine and into pre-modern times.[9] These instructions were later supported by Galen (130–c200) who also wrote and confirmed that venesection should be on the same side as the disease.[10] The reason being to drain bad blood from a vein situated close to the disease.

When the works of Aristotle, Hippocrates and Galen were translated from Greek into Arabic in the 9th century, the Muslim translator interpreted the texts to align them in accordance with the teachings of Islam. It was these texts that first reached the Western European Universities of Oxford, Paris and Cambridge in the 12th and 13th centuries after they had been translated into Latin. The point of interest here is that the Arab translations stated that venesection should take place on the opposite side from the 'bad blood'. The reason the translator changed sides is not clear and may have been an error or mistranslation.

The change to bleeding on the opposite side to the injury was made by Avicenna (980-1037). He was the most famous of the Arabic physicians and philosophers and was influential throughout the world of Islam and also Western Europe. He wrote that the blood vessel selected for venesection, 'in acute cases such as injuries or acute infections must be on the side away from the disease'.[11]

The West European University 'Scholastics', who are introduced in Chapter 10, had long since accepted Avicenna's interpretation. They could not know that copies of Hippocrates' and Galen's original texts had remained sequestered in the scriptoria of the Monasteries of Constantinople and Byzantium.

These original untranslated treatises were only rediscovered and transferred to Italy following the sack of Constantinople by the army of the 4th Crusade in 1204. These purely Greek texts direct from the monasteries were obviously without any Arabic interpretation. They were now translated directly from Greek into Latin by Italian scholars. These treatises confirmed that Hippocrates and Galen had written that venesection should be carried out on the same side as the wound or disease.

On account of the disagreement over which side venesection should take place, there then arose in 16th century Paris, a dispute between those who supported the 'Arabists' to bleed on the opposite side to the disease and those who were now following the rediscovered works of Hippocrates and Galen who stipulated venesection must be on the same side.

This dispute was so serious that it shook Christendom. The schism that now occurred had a far-reaching negative effect on the Scholastics[12] in the universities, for it was they who had always accepted the Arabist[13] interpretations of the Greek writings as sacrosanct. They had even made these texts part of the core curriculum of their universities.

In 1514, Dr Pierre Brissot (1478–1522), a learned professor in Paris, now conversant with a direct translation of Galen's work from Greek to Latin, immediately proclaimed that venesection should be practised on the same side as the disease in order to remove 'the fouled blood and to attract the good'.[14]

The ensuing conflict seems incredible. The French Parliament dealt with Brissot by banishing him from France. Meanwhile those agreeing with Brissot continued their opposition against the Arab version of the site for venesection. This row even reached the throne of Emperor Charles V,who then proclaimed Brissot to be 'as infamous as Martin Luther (1483-1546)'and Pope Clement VII joined in by agreeing with the Emperor.

In the midst of the argument, a relative of the Emperor died of pneumonia in one lung. The rumour grew that she had undergone venesection in the orthodox Arab tradition on the opposite side of the body and not on the same side as laid down by Galen. This threw everybody into confusion. The judgments of the Emperor and the Pope had been proved wrong. Many of Brissot's followers stopped practising venesection, except for Leonardo Botallo (1519–1587) and his school who turned 'vampire' and increased their frequency of venesections[15] while proclaiming that it should be practised on the same side.

This surreal farrago weakened the grip of the Scholastics' adherence to Galen's Arabist works in the universities. The initial effect was small due to their strong belief in their own 'stupefying and obsequious scholarship'. Although the dogma advocating venesection was weakened, the belief in it was so entrenched that it continued as before. It also needs to be taken into consideration that there was no other 'treatment' available, in those days before the causes of disease were known, but it did begin to register that the Greeks, the innovators and intellectual leaders in their own times were not omniscient after all.

The practice of venesection continued in Europe through to the early modern times. There is a report in England that Dr Matthew Baillie (1761–1823), a physician and nephew of Mr John Hunter (1728–1793), criticised and denounced the practice of venesection in 1817. For at this time, it had reached the height of its popularity with the development of multiple methods of administration. Those described in medical textbooks ranged from dry cupping, scarification, venesection, arteriotomy and the use of leeches. In fact, the breeding of leeches developed into an industry. Venesection continued thereafter mainly through the use of leeches and now cupping a mild successor is still in use in some countries.

In conclusion, the history of venesection is strange but gripping. Strange that a totally useless treatment should have been an essential part of medical practice for over 2300 years, albeit in an attenuated form in later years. Gripping, because both medical practitioners and their patients had accepted this 'treatment'. As already noted, the supposed proof of its success rested on the fact that most patients survived. It was a logical treatment when applying the Greek theory of disease before the actual causes of diseases were known.

Now the Ancient Greeks having freed themselves from superstition from the 6th century BC, then used their 'mind's eye' to theorise and produce a framework within which to practice medicine and surgery. It included the four humours with their associated equilibrium or disequilibrium before the dawn of science, at a time when their tools were few and knowledge of anatomy and physiology negligible.

It was also possible that many of the Ancient Greek manuscripts, philosophical as well as medical and surgical, might have been lost except for the diligence of the Arab scholars who translated them. Translating these works had been acceptable to them because they believed that the Greek philosophers were monotheists like themselves, albeit pagans. This enabled them to align Greek philosophy with the teachings of Islam. If on the other hand, the Greek philosophers had been considered polytheists, then their philosophy would not have been of interest and so not translated. Under these circumstances, the course of history and philosophy in medieval and early modern Western Europe might have been very different and more primitive as discussed in Chapter 13.

A harsh view of these times of conflict was forcefully expressed by Dr Majno who wrote in 1975. 'Europe sank into the Dark Ages...only the number of wounds did not decline, as I fear they will always be a basic means of human communication'.[16]

References:

1. *The Healing Hand. Man and Wound in the Ancient World.* By Guido Majno. Harvard University Press. 1975. p 129–130.
2. *The Healing Hand. Man and Wound in the Ancient World.* By Guido Majno. Harvard University Press. 1975. p 86.
3. *Hippocratic Writings.* Editor G.E.R. Lloyd. Penguin Books. 1950, reprinted 1983, p. 25 & 26.
4. *The Healing Hand. Man and Wound in the Ancient World.* By Guido Majno. Harvard University Press. 1985, p 181.
5. *Ditto.* P 182.
6. *Ditto.* P 178.
7. *Ditto.* P 180.
8. *Ditto.* P. 178.
9. *The Greeks.* By H. Kitto. Penguin History, 1991. Quotation of Charles Daremberg.
10. Hippocratic Writings. Edited by G.E.R. Lloyd. Penguin Books, 1983, p. 269.
11. *The Canon of Medicine.* By Avicenna. Adapted by Laleh Bakhtiar. Great Books of the Islamic World, Inc1999. p 511–512. And, Abū 'Alī al-Husayn ibn Abdullah ibn Sīna (983–1037) was known in the Latin West as Avicenna.
12. *Arabian Medicine and its Influence on the Middle Ages.* By Dr Donald Campbell. Pub. Kegan Paul, Trubner & Co. Ltd. London. 1926. P. 155.
13. Ibid., P. 165–166.
14. *The Historical Relations of medicine and Surgery to the End of the Sixteenth Century. An Address Delivered at the St Louis Congress in 1904.* Allbutt, T. Clifford (1836–1925). Macmillan and Co. New York, 1905, p 107.
15. *The Historical Relations of medicine and Surgery to the End of the Sixteenth Century. An Address Delivered at the St Louis Congress in 1904.* Allbutt, T. Clifford (1836–1925). Macmillan and Co. New York, 1905, 107–108.
16. *The Healing Hand. Man and Wound in the Ancient World.* By Guido Majno. Harvard University Press. 1985, p 417.

Chapter 8
Analysis of Surgery in the Second Period

1. The Ancient Greeks dominate surgical practice.
2. Surgery in Homer's time.
3. Original operations undertaken by the Ancient Greeks.
4. The Greeks provide medical and surgical services in the Roman Empire.
5. India's contribution to original operations.
6. No original operations were produced in Byzantium.
7. Analysis of all the original operations from, Egypt, Ancient Greece and India.
8. Ancient Chinese surgery.
9. Summary.

1. The Ancient Greeks dominate surgical practice.

The Ancient Greek dominance in medicine and surgery was an unbroken continuum beginning in the City States of Greece with Hippocrates in the 5th century BC; it continued during the brief Empire of Alexander the Great and the subsequent division of his empire. It later survived the fall of Athens and then all of Greece to the armies of the Roman Republic. It was then that Greek doctors migrated to Rome and became the principal providers of medical and surgical services there. Then when the Roman Empire declined in the West, it brought an end to this extraordinary period of Ancient Greek surgical ingenuity. It is then notable that the Greek speaking Byzantine Empire, formerly the Eastern Roman Empire, with its capital in Constantinople produced no original operations.

A smaller Indian contribution of five original operations had been separately developed in about the 2nd century BC. These were all sophisticated operations. The overall complexity of operations during this second period of surgery demonstrates a considerable leap forward beyond the achievements of the Ancient Egyptians.

There were many factors that led to the Greek intellectual dominance. Among these was the geography of Greece with its mountainous terrain enclosing fertile valleys. This physical isolation of each territory favoured the formation of small city states, that maintained their independence for only about four centuries. During this critical time, especially in Athens, they governed themselves by assemblies of their citizens. This short period was long enough for them to exercise their genius for independent thought.

The citizens of these city states elected magistrates from amongst themselves and collectively made political decisions for war or peace. When they decided that war was necessary, it was the citizens themselves who voted for it and they themselves took up arms and put themselves at risk. Matters of common interest were fiercely debated and different sides of an argument were heard before decisions were agreed. Within this novel environment, the citizens thought for themselves. This was quite unlike people who lived under the autocratic rule of kings or emperors, who demanded blind obedience from their subjects. It was this independence of thought that enabled the Greeks to develop not only philosophy, but also their theories of medicine and surgery.

An important factor enabling the Greek City States to develop during this period was that they were undisturbed by attacks from foreign enemies. It was an unusual time for the kings and empires surrounding them were either developing or in a weakened state.

Another advantage for the Greeks was the high level of literacy among the citizens. Initially, this was due to peripatetic teachers who travelled from city to city teaching reading and writing, but they also began to teach philosophy and governance. The Greek language itself enabled the expression of abstract thought, so intellectual ideas and concepts could be formulated, discussed and developed. The nature of the Greek language is to express accurately not only the relationship between ideas but also shades of meaning, as the nature of the language is to be exact. This led to the development of schools, such as the School of Medicine on the island of Cos where Hippocrates practised medicine and wrote his treatises. These were not schools in the modern sense, but places where those who were like-minded could learn, formulate and advance ideas and they are probably best thought of as the forerunners of universities.

It was within this intellectual[1] atmosphere that Plato (c428–348 BC) arrived in Athens in about 388 BC and founded the Academy. It rapidly acquired intellectual and educational leadership of the Greek world that lasted three hundred years in the first instance. This ended at the beginning of the 1st century BC when Athens was sacked by the Romans.

Plato's Academy was the model for the Museum and Library in Alexandria in Egypt founded in about 307 BC. The Museum and Library, in various forms, lasted for over nine hundred years and became in turn the main Hellenistic centre for philosophy and scientific research, that continued as a centre of intellectual advancement after it was incorporated into the Roman Empire. It was in Alexandria that anatomy and physiology were first systematically studied and demonstrated.

One of Plato's students at the Academy was Aristotle of Stagira (384–322 BC) who remained there for twenty years. After Plato's death, Aristotle travelled in Asia Minor and then stayed for a time on the Island of Lesbos; there he applied himself to the study of natural history, a subject considered by other philosophers of that time as being unworthy of attention because it concerned 'the corporeal and not the intellectual world'.

Aristotle's treatise *Historia Animalium*[2] was the first of its kind and describes his observations and dissections of hundreds of insects, fish, birds and mammals. He considered each a species and for groups of similar creatures, he was moving towards the concept of a genus. The more he studied, the greater his understanding of the variety, yet similarity of life. He made comparisons of locomotion, the brain, digestion, the respiratory system and reproduction. His aim was not only to discover facts, 'That things are so', but to reveal causes, 'How and why they are so,' and thereby to reveal the absence of chance in works of nature. The ideas Aristotle expressed were revolutionary and represent the beginning of natural science and later the study of human anatomy. In 342 BC, Aristotle accepted an invitation to tutor Alexander, later the Great. He returned to Athens in 335 BC and founded a new school, the Lyceum, that became another intellectual powerhouse and where he remained at its Head for the rest of his life.

After his death, Alexander-the-Great's (356–323 BC) empire was divided among his generals. His former General Ptolemy[3] ruled Egypt between 323 BC and 284 BC by founding the last dynasty of the Pharaohs. It was Ptolemy, who being interested in philosophy and medicine built the Museum and Library in Alexandria. Within twenty years of its foundation, the Museum in Alexandria had become famous as a school where Greek scholars actively pursued many aspects of what we now know as science including the study of human anatomy and physiology. It was probably the world's first university.

Of particular note among the scholars was Herophilos of Chalcedon (335–280 BC) and Erasistratus[4&5] of Ceos (c304–c250 BC). Herophilos[6] was the first to carry out systematic human dissections that were permitted during the reign of the second Ptolemy. He also followed Aristotle's idea in considering it essential to base knowledge on an empirical basis. He gave specific names to some anatomical organs, such as the duodenum.

Erasistratus also advanced anatomy through human dissection and discovered the one-way function of the valves in the heart. These early anatomists made a tentative start of unravelling the anatomy and functioning of the body. During this period, other technical advances were also made, including the development of the syringe and pump by Ctesibius (285–222 BC).[7] The intellectual output of the Greeks continued to grow through their schools of learning, where experiments in the science of surgery were actively pursued. All these developments provided the conditions conducive to the production of original operations.

To fully appreciate the work of those who have made discoveries in the past, whether in philosophy, early science or surgery, it is essential and necessary to compare their work with that of their predecessors and not with their successors. Using this interpretation, the Ancient Greeks demonstrated an unprecedented intellectual advance compared to the past.

2. Surgery in Homer's time.

After outlining the background for the intellectual development of the Ancient Greeks, a brief look at surgery in Homer's time gives a comparison with what was to follow.

In the *Odyssey*, written about 800 BC, Homer gives the first example of the attitude to treatment of wounds in Greek literature. His description of the blinding of Cyclops' single eye was followed by Odysseus calmly saying, 'Sickness comes from almighty Zeus and cannot be helped. All you can do is pray'...[8]

This was a resigned approach caused by the lack of any therapy, at a time when such matters were considered to be purely in the lap of the gods.

This contrasts with Homer's 'Iliad', when Machaon after being wounded in the right shoulder by a three barbed arrow is being encouraged to seek treatment with the words, 'A leech is worth many other men, to cut out arrows, and spread soothing medicaments'.[9]

This was practical surgery, similar to that found in the Edwin Smith papyrus of 1,700 BC and despite the archaic language, hints at a respect for surgeons.

3. Original operations undertaken by the Ancient Greeks.

Five original operations are attributed to Hippocrates as shown in Box 8.1. One of these is the attribution for bladder-stone excision through a perineal incision. It has been unclear in the past to whom this operation should be attributed, either to the Hindu physician and surgeon Sushruta[10]
or to Hippocrates. Sushruta wrote a description of how to carry out this operation. However, the excision of bladder stones has been included here among the works of Hippocrates for the following reason.

Bladder stones were common in antiquity and through to the late Middle Ages. Hippocrates gives a command to new physicians and surgeons in the 'Oath' that they swore before beginning their independent careers. In it, he writes, 'I will not cut, even for the stone, but will leave such procedures to the practitioners of the craft'.[11&12]

Hippocrates was well-aware of the operation and the probable reason for his caution was the high mortality of over 50% of those who underwent it.

BOX 8. 1

TWENTY-EIGHT ORIGINAL OPERATIONS FROM THE SECOND PERIOD, ALL OF ANCIENT GREEK AND INDIAN ORIGIN.

HIPPOCRATES	**UNKNOWN**	**SUSHRUTA**
460-370 BC	**c320 BC**	**c200 BC**
Fistula-in-ano[14]	Caesarean section[17]	Surgery snakebites[18]
Haemorrhoidectomy[40]		Earlobe reconstruction[19]
Excision of dead foetus[15]		Nasal reconstruction[20]
Venesection[13]		Couching cataracts[21]
Bladder stone excision[16]		

CELSUS		
c25-c50 AD		
Ligation of arteries[22]	Amputations[23]	Tonsilectomy[24]
Umbilical hernia[25]	Inguinal hernia[26]	Varicocele[27]
Varicose veins[28]	Urethral stones[29]	Colonic suture[30]
Circumcision reversal[31]	Abdominal ascites[32]	Partial-thyroidectomy[33]
Mastectomy[34]	Hydrocele[35]	

SORANUS	**ANTYLLUS**	**GALEN**
c120 AD	**c170 AD**	**130-200 AD**
Vaginal-Hysterectomy[36]	Ligation of aneurysm[38]	Suturing muscles and tendons[37]
	Tracheostomy[39]	

The practitioners he refers to were generally itinerants, often families who passed the technique from one generation to the next. They escaped each town for fear of retribution when their high mortality became apparent. Bladder stones are usually caused by precipitation of magnesium and calcium salts in a bladder that cannot completely empty, usually due to an enlarged prostate.

The controversy over the primacy for this original operation has involved both Indian and European scholars and arose from the difficulty of accurately dating Sushruta's writings. For millennia, India had an oral tradition of passing on knowledge and dates were not recorded. This resulted in the difficulty of giving a date for when Sushruta was actively in practice. The most recent study concerning the date of his book, the *Sushruta Samhita*, has placed his writing at about 200 BC,[41] giving Hippocrates claim to have been the first to record this operation by nearly 200 years. Should cogent new evidence be produced this date may need to be revised, but weather it is a Greek or Indian original operation will not affect its inclusion.

One of Hippocrates' greatest contributions to medicine was his declaration that disease was caused by natural phenomena and not inflicted on humans as a punishment or due to the caprice of the gods. This entirely new concept enabled him and his successors to seek a framework of how disease was caused. This was in sharp contrast to the beliefs of the Ancient Egyptians and Homer. Hippocrates' system enabled the Ancient Greek physicians and surgeons and their successors to practise consistently within an intellectual framework, as has been described in earlier chapters. Hippocrates' system was so successful that it went unchallenged for over 2300 years and only became obsolete when the actual causes of diseases were discovered.

Hippocrates kept careful medical records over a long period of time, enabling him to recognise the progress of individual diseases. As a result, he was often able to give his patients a diagnosis and also a prognosis that added to his fame. His high moral principles were instilled in his students by demanding from them 'decorum, probity and honesty' in their practice of medicine. His oath has been sworn since the early 5th century BC and was still being sworn by newly qualified doctors receiving their degrees in the 20th century; amongst them was the author in the 1960s.

Hippocratic surgery was more complex than that of the Ancient Egyptians who had laid the foundations for the practice of surgery by developing the original-procedures of catheterisation, suturing, setting of bones and reduction of dislocations, all of which continued to be practised by the Ancient Greeks and also by surgeons ever since. None of the ancients operated electively within the great cavities of the body. In those days if the peritoneal cavity had been opened in battle or in a fight, then death was almost inevitable due to sepsis.

Unsurprisingly, the old beliefs and practices of healing did not suddenly cease because of this new philosophy of medicine and surgery. They continued in competition with it, in the temples, especially those dedicated to the Greek god Asclepius.

4. The Greeks provide medical and surgical services in the Roman Empire.

Greek philosophy was much admired by educated Romans. Their interest started before the beginning of their conquest of Greece, that began with the fall of Corinth in 146 BC and was finally accomplished when Athens fell in 88 BC.

It was after this that many Greek physicians and surgeons migrated to practise within the Roman Republic and then Empire.

The relationship of the Romans to the Greeks is interesting. Broadly speaking, the Roman elite were politicians, soldiers, administrators and engineers. The Greeks provided the Empire with philosophers, teachers and practitioners of medicine and surgery. To be a physician, at a time when physicians were also surgeons, was beneath the dignity of a Roman. In this, they differed from the Greeks for whom medicine and surgery were honourable occupations and undertaken by the most educated of men. It is not therefore surprising that Greek physicians made their way to Rome and the other great cities of the Empire to practise. They also enlisted as military surgeons to the Legions. Their services were generally appreciated and Greeks rose to be physicians to Roman Emperors. The most famous medical school during the Roman Empire continued to be the Library and Museum in Alexandria in Egypt, where Greek was still the language used, even after Egypt had been annexed to Rome in 30 BC.

Aulus Celsus[42] (c25 BC–c50 AD), a Roman citizen born in what is now France, spent most of his life in Rome where he wrote eight books on medicine and surgery that have survived. He also wrote extensively on agriculture, military arts, rhetoric, philosophy and jurisprudence. He was the only well-known author of medical and surgical treatises in ancient times who wrote in Latin rather than Greek. In his medical treatises, he records 14 original operations listed in Box 8.1 above. Whether Celsus was a physician and surgeon has not been established. He certainly was an encyclopaedist. The evidence for this comes from another Roman encyclopaedist, Gaius Pliny the Elder[42] (23–79 AD), who was a contemporary of Celsus and described him as an author and not a physician. Pliny died in the eruption of Mount Vesuvius in 79 AD.

The fact that documents in Greek were translated by Celsus into Latin also confirms that medicine and surgery in the Roman Empire was a continuation of the Ancient Greek practice. For the purposes of this book, all operations described by Celsus are for simplicity attributed to him. He performed a great service by preserving the knowledge of so many Ancient Greek original operations that may well have been otherwise lost. It is also of note that he was the first to translate Greek philosophy, medicine and surgery into Latin. His writings reached Western Europe much later than those of Hippocrates and Galen and were eventually published in Florence in 1478.[43] His descriptions of

14 original operations significantly increased the known numbers undertaken and identified as of Greek origin. Technically, only one of these operations took place within the abdominal cavity and that was in a man whose abdomen had been slashed open in conflict.

This needs further comment, for any wound in which the abdomen was laid open and the bowel pierced, almost inevitably resulted in death due to peritonitis. Under these circumstances, suturing the colon and closure of the abdomen was rarely successful. Such an operation must have been an emergency procedure, but does not represent the beginning of elective abdominal surgery, for that had to wait until 1809.[44 43] Celsus confirmed the poor outcome in such cases. One hopes he was gratified with the result and that his patient survived, for we are not told. He was the first to report the practice of tying bleeding arteries. This was life-saving following wounds in battle and those received by gladiators. It was indeed the first step in vascular surgery. For before this innovation, a haemorrhaging artery was usually treated by red-hot cautery frequently with disastrous results.

He described surgery as that part of the, 'Art of medicine that cures by hand and the effects of this treatment are more obvious than any other kind'. His description of an ideal surgeon states he should have a 'strong and steady hand; with vision sharp and clear, and spirit undaunted; filled with pity, so he wishes to cure the patient, but is not moved by his cries'.[45 44] It is salutary for a modern surgeon to try to imagine what it must have been like to operate while patients screamed throughout the operation while being constrained by strong men, these difficulties inevitably limited the range of surgery possible before anaesthesia. Surgeons did not operate within the great body cavities and were restricted to the superficial tissues. This includes the operation for bladder stones, that was accomplished through a perineal incision close to the anus and did not enter the peritoneal cavity.

Usually, an operation would only last a minute or two, as with amputations. The longest recorded was just under 30 minutes, for very few could tolerate the pain for this length of time. Professor Harold Ellis tells us in, *Operations that Made History,* how before anaesthesia Sir Astley Cooper[46] in 1824 carried out a disarticulation of the femur in just under half an hour in a stoical patient. Returning to the Greeks, Celsus recognised the importance of anatomy to the practice of surgery and wrote, 'as pains and also various kinds of diseases arise in the more internal parts, they hold that no-one can apply remedies for these, who is ignorant about the parts themselves'.[47 46] He was referring to internal anatomy that was then a mystery.

After Celsus, Soranus of Ephesus[48] (fl c120 AD) another Greek surgeon in the time of the Roman Empire, performed the first vaginal hysterectomy where he saved a woman's life by excising a gangrenous prolapsed uterus with success.[47]

In about 170 AD, Antyllus[49] (f c170 AD) undertook two original operations in Rome. These were treatment for an aneurysm of the brachial artery at the elbow, when he ligated the artery above the aneurysm so prevented it from rupturing. His other original operation, at about the same time, was a tracheostomy that was formerly attributed to Paul of Aegina in the 6th century. Paul gives a good description of a tracheostomy that he carried out as a successor surgeon.

The most famous of the Romano-Greek physicians and surgeons was Claudius Galen[50] (130–c200 AD). A Roman citizen, born in Pergamon in Asia Minor of a well-to-do Greek father who gave him an exemplary education. He became the greatest anatomist of his day studying first in Corinth and Smyrna and he then spent several years in Alexandria in Egypt. There he performed meticulous dissections on barbary apes,[51] using them as a proxy for humans, since human dissection was forbidden by the Roman authorities. His book, *Anatomical Procedures,* along with his surgical writings were serially translated from Greek into Syriac, Arabic, Latin and finally the vernacular languages of Europe. He also carried out the first true physiological experiments. Galen's experience of surgery was impressive; for several years, he was surgeon to the gladiators in Pergamon and then served as a military surgeon for five years with a Roman Legion. He was later appointed physician to Commodus, the son of the Emperor Marcus Aurelius.

In 177, Galen retired from public life to practise and lecture in Rome, always speaking and writing in Greek. His detailed anatomical lectures are easy to read. In all, he produced ten books on anatomy and altogether wrote two million words covering philosophy and many other subjects as well as medicine and surgery. He also laid the foundations for further advances in surgery and wrote that experiments should continue. This particular advice was ignored when his book *On Anatomical Procedures* along with his other surgical writings were later translated into Arabic. The study of practical anatomy hardly progressed after his death until the 16th century. It had to wait until Vesalius had re-established the study of anatomy.

Before this time, Galen's treatises on anatomy and surgery[52] were the textbooks that were consulted as the definitive authority on these subjects for the next 1300 years, in Rome, Byzantium, the Arab Empires, Italy and finally Western Europe.

Surprisingly, Galen only developed one original operation, which was the primary suturing of tendons and nerves after they had been severed in gladiatorial contests or battle. It was a puzzle why the greatest surgeon of his time, whose works became standard textbooks up to the end of the medieval era, only devised a single original operation. The reason for this will become clear in due course.

It is also worth mentioning that the Roman military were the first to design and build hospitals.[53] From about 79 AD, they built over 20 hospitals that could accommodate 200 wounded or sick soldiers. These hospitals were spacious and well planned and built along the frontiers of the Empire from Scotland to Syria. Each hospital or 'valetudinarium' was largely staffed by Greek surgeons.

5. India's contribution to original operations.

The first recorded Caesarean section was carried out in India in c320 BC. The baby who was delivered by this operation was Bindusara, who became the second Mauryan Emperor of India. A caesarean section in those days would only be possible in the household of a king or emperor with a surgeon to hand with appropriate instruments and a valuable heir to be delivered.[54]

The subsequent Indian contribution to this second period was remarkable. In about 200 BC, four original operations were described by Sushruta. He was the founder of plastic surgery with two operations. One was a pedicle graft to repair ruptured earlobes, an injury that was not uncommon amongst Brahmins who wore heavy earrings that pulled down on the loop of the ear and not infrequently ruptured it.[55] Sushruta's reconstruction was described in terms that could be followed by a modern surgeon.[54] He was also the first to describe nasal reconstructions,[56] using a skin flap from the forehead. He was also responsible for the first invasive operation on the eye, by couching cataracts[57] [56] and he described surgical treatment for snakebites that included the use of a tourniquet.[58]

Like Hippocrates, Sushruta's writings are not the work of one man and were likely to have accumulated over a period of time. He attracted disciples who followed and worked with him in an informal arrangement. As already mentioned, he does not seem to have left a theory or philosophy of surgery.

6. No original operations were produces in Byzantium

Box 8.2.[59]

Operations practised in Byzantium 200 to 660. None were original operations.

1. Use of ligatures.
2. Hernia ops.
3. Incision of abscesses.
4. Operations for fistulae.
5. Circumcision.
6. Hydrocele excision.
7. Excision urethral stones.
8. Haemorrhoidectomy.
9. Varicose vein ops.
10. Excision of dead foetus.
11. Mastectomy.
12. Venesection.
13. Trephination of skull.
14. Setting of fractures.
15. Reduction of dislocations.
16. Paracentesis for ascites.
17. Couching of cataracts.
18. Aneurysmal surgery.
19. Tracheostomy.

Claudius Galen (130–c200 AD) was the last of the Greek Romans to undertake an original operation in about 180. Medicine and surgery in the Empire went into steep decline and following the sacking of Rome in 410 were forgotten in Italy and in all the former Roman provinces in the west, including England. It has already been noted that under the Saxons,[60] surgery declined to the primitive level of incising abscesses and little else a situation that did not **to** improve until the Middle Ages.

The new ruler, Alaric the Goth (394-410) was so enamoured of the institutions of the Roman empire that he maintained them, after settling one third of the former Roman lands on his followers. Among the institutions he cherished was the Roman Catholic Church that in time converted the Goths. The relevance of this to surgery will become apparent in later chapters.

Meanwhile, Byzantium the former Eastern Roman Empire was not affected and continued to function normally, but developed into a rigid theocracy that actively discouraged free thought and re-embraced the idea that disease was divine punishment for sins. Guided by religious orthodoxy and both distracted and occupied by trying to retake the Western Roman Empire from the Goths and Visigoths during the next century, medicine and surgery were neglected and no further original operations were undertaken. Not only that, but the Library in

Alexandria in Egypt was ransacked on the orders of the Emperor Justinian (482-565) to destroy philosophic Greek treatises that he considered to be heretical, especially those of Plato and Aristotle.

Surgery had now entered a long period during which no original operations took place. This included not only Byzantium, but also the Arab Empires and finally the Middle Ages in Europe until the mid-16th century and so this period lasted for a staggering 1300 years. There were common causes for this absence of original operations as well as different reasons specific to each of them that will be described later. Looking at this second period alone, the reasons for the lack of original operations can be attributed to two main causes which are discussed in the next section.

Meanwhile, in Byzantium, the monasteries used their scriptoria to copy the treatises of Hippocrates, Plato, Aristotle and Galen. Some of these documents were transferred to Alexandria in Egypt, others taken to Syria by the Nestorians[61] following their expulsion from Byzantium in 431 AD, while other copies remained lodged in the monastic libraries of Byzantium, where they remained untouched until Constantinople was sacked by the soldiers of the Fourth Crusade on their way to the Holy Land in 1204.

Apart from a short period of time in Alexandria when human dissection was allowed, it was otherwise forbidden on religious grounds. After Galen's death, the lack of attention to anatomy also led to the end of the experimental physiology which he had both developed and excelled. No such pursuit of knowledge took place in Byzantium, but it did boost Galens[62] legacy in medieval times.

The result was that Galen's anatomy of apes and descriptions of Greek original operations became the final and definitive source of information for the practice of surgery into the 18th century. One imagines that Galen himself would have expected physiological experiments and advances in surgery to progress, rather than that his works came to be quoted as the last word in surgery and anatomy for nearly 1300 years.[62]

These were the main contributory reasons for the cessation of original operations in Byzantium.

7. Analysis of all the original operations from, Egypt, Ancient Greece and India.

Figure 8.1, shows all the original operations and procedures developed during the Egyptian and Greek periods of surgery, that ended in or before 200. This date marked the end of the Greek period of original operations. Adding the 23 Greek and five Indian original operations to the earlier eight, from Peru and ancient Egypt amounts to a considerable legacy of 36 generic original operations.

These ancient surgeons extensively operated on and were almost completely limited to operating on the superficial tissues of the body. It remained the case, that with only one exception, no planned operations were undertaken within the brain, thorax or abdomen until after the advent of anaesthesia. To be included as an original operation, patients must be able to benefit from the operation and survive, even though many did die from post-operative complications, of which septicaemia was the commonest.

Surgery was then often only carried out when the patient knew that death was inevitable without it. Among these operations were strangulated hernias, loss of consciousness due to intracranial bleeding and the necessity for an urgent tracheostomy due to respiratory obstruction. The risk of bladder stone surgery was accepted by patients when the pain was persistent and unbearable. Other life and death operations included snakebites and ligations of bleeding arteries to prevent exsanguination. Many operations were undertaken, then as now, due to conditions that stopped patients from working, such as gross haemorrhoids and anal fistulae. Some were emergencies such as a caesarean section to save a baby usually with the tragic death of the mother. Some operations were cosmetic as with the ear lobe and nasal reconstructions of Sushruta, the beginning of plastic surgery.

The one exception to entering the abdomen was the suturing of a lacerated colon following abdominal trauma[63] that was described by Celsus. Surgeons at that time were well aware that opening the peritoneal cavity was usually followed by peritonitis and death.

The extraordinary fact is that all these operations and more had been written down and described in detail. Figure 8.1, shows how comprehensively the superficial tissues of the body had been operated upon by 180 AD.

Figure 8.1.

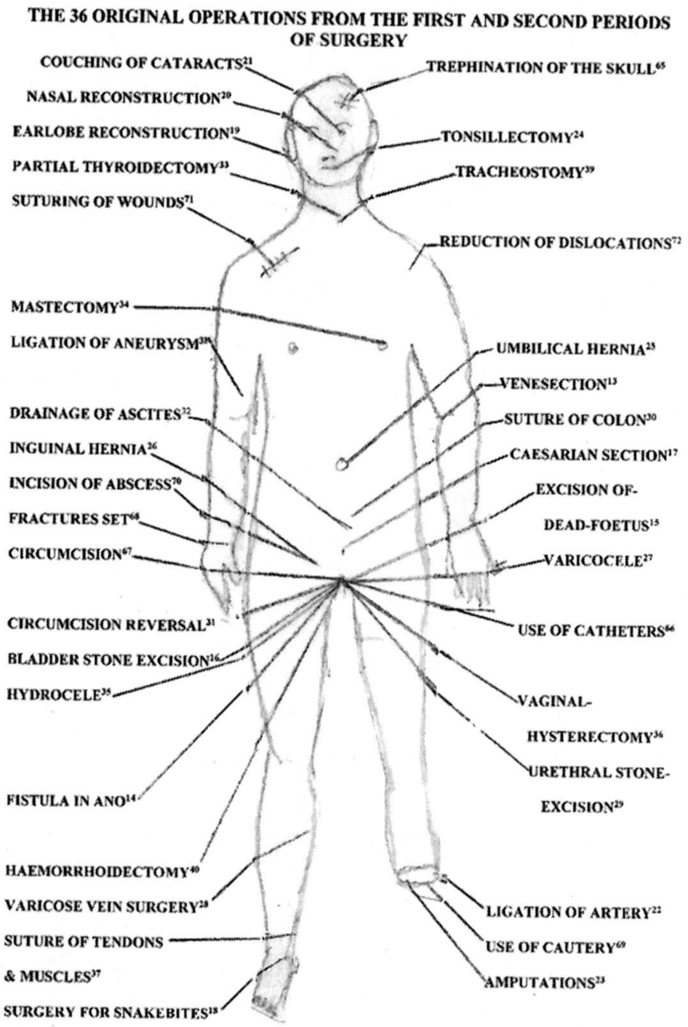

8. Ancient Chinese surgery.

The Chinese contribution to surgery during this same period was disappointing. Surgery was considered a lowly occupation in China while physicians were well respected. Guido Majno in *The Healing Hand*[64] informs us that the Chinese list five kinds of treatment, 'psychological, dietary, drugs, acupuncture and clinical medicine'. Surgeons are hardly mentioned and were not given the respect that Hindu and Greek surgeons received.

At about the same time that Hippocrates was active, a search revealed only one recorded operation in China. This operation was not to treat disease, but to castrate men to turn them into eunuchs by excising their male organs. This operation had been practiced from antiquity into the early 20th century but ceased with the fall of the last Emperor in 1912. Castration has not been included among the original operations, as it was not performed to relieve disease or suffering. The operation to amputate all the genitals was accomplished with a single sweep of a sickle shaped knife.

9. Summary.

This second period of original operations represents the first flowering of surgery by the Ancient Greeks and Sushruta's operations from India. Greek genius for independent thought and their development of philosophy, medicine and surgery were born in the freedom of the City States. These lasted long enough for independent thought to be established. As a result, the philosophy of the Ancients along with medicine and surgery, survived the destruction of the Academy and Lyceum in Athens by the Romans, and later the Library and Museum in Alexandria in Egypt. These centres of learning had stimulated and passed on the works of Hippocrates, Galen and others as a continuum and they were not surpassed until the late medieval and early modern periods. The first Golden Age of innovation in surgery, demonstrated by the original operations described, had now ended.

References:

1. *Plato. Ancient Culture and Society: Early Greek Science. G.E.R. Lloyd, Chapter Eight.*
2. *The Works of Aristotle Translated into English. Vol. IV. Historia Animalium, By D'Arcy Wentworth Thompson. Clarendon Press, Oxford. 1910.*
3. Wikipedia. Ptolomy 1 Soter of Eqypt. Eristatratus.

4. *The Heart and Vascular System in Ancient Greek Medicine. From Alcmaeon to Galen.* By C R. S. Harris. Oxford, Clarendon Press. 1983 p 224 & 378. Erasistratus.
5. As in 4.
6. *Herophilus of Calcedon.* Chapter 2. Circa 320 BC.
7. Ctesibus. Chapter 2, c250 BC.
8. *The Odyssey.* Homer, translated by E.V. Rieu. Guild Publishing, London, 1988. p 150.
9. *The Iliad of Homer.* Translated by Andrew Lang, Walter Leaf and Ernest Myers. Publisher Macmillan & Co Ltd, London. 1912. p 218.
10. *Hippocratic Writings.* Edited by G.E.R. Lloyd. Penguin Classics Reprinted 1983 ISBN 13: 988-0-14-044451-3. p 67. Bladder stones.
11. Hippocrates Oath. In Hippocratic Writing. G.E.R. Lloyd. Page 67.
12. As in 11.
13. Chapter 2. c425 BC, Venesection.
14. Ibid. c425 BC, Fistula-in-ano.
15. Ibid. c425 BC Excision of dead foetus.
16. Ibid. c425 BC. Excision of bladder stones.
17. Ibid. c320 BC. Caesarean section.
18. Ibid. c200 BC. Snake bites.
19. Ibid. c200 BC. Earlobe reconstruction.
20. Ibid. c200 BC. Nasal reconstruction.
21. Ibid. c200 BC. Couching cataracts.
22. Ibid. c30 AD. Ligation of arteries.
23. Ibid. c30 AD. Amputations.
24. Ibid. c30 AD. Tonsillectomy.
25. Ibid. c30 AD. Umbilical hernia.
26. Ibid. c30 AD. Inguinal hernia.
27. Ibid. c30 AD. Excision of varicocele.
28. Ibid. c30 AD. Varicose veins.
29. Ditto. c30 AD. Excision of urethral stone.
30. Ditto. c30 AD. Suturing of colon.
31. Ditto. c30 AD. Reversal of circumcision.
32. Ditto. c30 BC. Drainage of ascites.
33. Ditto. c30 BC. Partial thyroidectomy.
34. Ditto. c30 BC. Mastectomy.

35. Ditto. c25 BC. Excision of hydrocele.
36. *Soranus's Gynaecology.* Translated by Owsei Temkin. The Johns Hopkins Press, Baltimore, USA, 1991. And vaginal hysterectomy, p 200–201. And Chapter 5. c120 AD.
37. Chapter 2. c79 AD. Suturing muscles and tendons.
38. Ibid. c170. Ligation of an aneurysm.
39. Ibid. c170. Tracheostomy.
40. Ibid. c425 BC. Haemorrhoidectomy.
41. *Dermatological writings of ancient India.* Menon I.A, Haberman H.F., (1969) Med. Hist. 13(4): 387–392. Sushruta
42. *Celsus on Medicine. Vol. 1, Book 1.* Translated by W.G. Spencer. Loeb Classical Library, Harvard University Press, 1935. Introduction by Dr W.H.S. Jones, p. VIII.
43. *The Legacy of Rome.* Edited by Cyril Bailey, Oxford at the Clarendon Press, reprinted in 1940. Chapter on Science by Charles Singer, p 284–285.
44. Chapter 2. 1809.
45. *Celsus on Medicine.* Loeb Classical Library, Harvard University Press, Books 7–8. 1938. p 297. The ideal surgeon.
46. *Operations that made History.* By Harold Ellis. Cambridge University Press. 2009, pp 24–25. Disarticulation of the femur.
47. *Celsus on Medicine. Loeb Classical Library Vol. 1, Book 1.* Harvard University Press, 1935. Introduction by Dr W. G. Spencer, pp 15, 17. Importance of anatomy.
48. Chapter 2. c120 AD. Soranus.
49. Ibid. c170 AD. Antyllus.
50. Ibid. c180 AD. Galen.
51. *Galen on Anatomical Procedures.* Translation of the surviving books with introduction and notes, by Charles Singer. Oxford University Press. Special Edition for Sandpiper Books, 1999.
52. Chapter 2. c180 AD, Galen sections 2, 3 & 4.
53. Ibid. c79 AD. Roman hospitals.
54. Ibid. c320 BC. Caesarean section.
55. Ibid. c200 BC. Sushruta. Earlobe reconstruction
56. Ibid. c200 BC. No. 2, Nasal reconstruction.
57. Ibid. c200 BC. Couching of cataracts No. 4.

58. Ibid. c200 BC. Snake bites, No. 1.
59. Operations practised in Byzantium. 200 to 660.
60. *General Medical Practice in Anglo-Saxon England.* By Wilfred Bonsor. Science Medicine and History, Essays on the Evolution of Scientific Thought and Medical Practice. Written in honour of Charles Singer. Vol. 1. p 154.
61. Chapter 2. c431 AD. Nestorius.
62. Ibid. c180 AD. Galen.
63. Ibid. c200 BC. Suturing of a perforated colon.
64. *The Healing Hand; Man and Wound in the Ancient World.* By Guido Majno. Harvard University Press, Cambridge Massachusetts, USA. Paperback edition 1991. ISBN. 0-674-38331-1. p 247–256.

Chapter 9: The Third Period

642 - 1084. The Arabian Empires.

The Preservation of Ancient Learning

The Byzantine Empire and Arabian Empires, and the transmission of Greek Manuscripts to Western Europe

1. The Arabian contribution to surgery.
2. Explanation for the absence of original operations during this period.
3. The transfer of Greek philosophy of surgery to Western Europe.

Box 9.1

The operations practiced in the Caliphates of Baghdad were all Egyptian, Ancient Greek and Indian original operations certainly some of them were practised.[17]

1. Incision of abscesses.[1]
2. Bladder stone excisions.[2]
3. Venesection.[3]
4. Reduction of dislocations.[4]
5. Setting of bone fracture.[5]
6. Tonsillectomy.[6]
7. Couching of cataracts.[7]
8. Circumcision.[8]
9. Trephination of the skull.[9]
10. Inguinal hernias.[10]
11. Haemorrhoidectomy.[11]
12. Amputation of the leg.[12]
    Some evidence for practise of the following:
13. Fistula-in-ano.[13]
14. Hydroceles.[14]
15. Closure of abdomen.[15]
16. Tracheostomy.[16]

1. The Arabian contribution to surgery

The Arabian Caliphates[17] valuable contribution to this history, developed through their interest in Greek philosophy. By translating Greek manuscripts into Arabic, they preserved the literature on medicine and surgery and also by aligning their translations to Islam, they took over the ownership of these texts as their own.[18]

This was later followed by two unexpected and unforeseeable consequences. First, it preserved for posterity the Greek manuscripts concerning philosophy and also, their theory and practice of surgery.

Second, the later translations of the manuscripts from Arabic into Latin that took place in Salerno in Italy and Toledo in Spain, kept their alignment with Islam.[19]

These Arabised Latin documents later became a template for European scholars of the 12th and 13th centuries to use in their turn. For they in turn realigned the philosophy of Plato and Aristotle from Islam to Christianity. By this process over a long period of time, they succeeded in separating religion from the science of the Ancient Greeks, especially that of Aristotle. The separation of these disciplines was not immediately accepted by the Catholic Church.[20] But by the 13th century, scientific experiments began to take place with the aim of exploring the workings of the corporeal or physical world.

To continue the speculation, it seems highly probable that this gradual separation of science from religion led to the much earlier development of science in Western Europe, than might otherwise have occurred. For the Arabic translations aligned with Islam were the template for introducing Christianity in its place. Taking this hypothesis a stage further, if this sequence of events had not taken place the gradual separation of religion from science may not have occurred or have been delayed by centuries. For the practice of science and development of technology was the stimulus that enabled an original operation to be undertaken in 1575 for the first time in one-thousand-three-hundred years. These matters are further discussed in due course.

2. A new explanation for the absence of original operations during this period.

The value of the Greek manuscripts can be judged by the time and effort that was expended on these translations by successive civilisations. This progression could have been disrupted by war or sheer disinterest at any time, as happened following the fall of Rome. The result there was that in the former Western Roman Empire, surgery regressed to a primitive state and did not even begin to improve for six centuries. None of this could have been predicted.

Meanwhile, a Golden Age was taking place in the Arabic Caliphates, centred in Baghdad and Cordova, with significant advances in astronomy, alchemy, mathematics, engineering, pharmacology and indeed medicine but not in surgery. For despite the flourishing of these other disciplines, surgeons did not undertake any original operations in this period, which has for a long time been an unexpected and puzzling anomaly.

I believe the explanation is that the original operations on the superficial tissues of the body, as described in Chapter 5, had already taken to its limits the organisation, technology and capabilities of the Ancient Egyptians, Greeks and Indians. The result was to leave no opportunity for the surgeons of the Arabian

Empires to undertake any original operations. It must be emphasised that there had not been any original operations after the end of the second period. For Byzantium, the former Eastern Roman Empire had not produced any after the fall of Rome and loss of the Western Empire. Then during the time of the Caliphates, this lack of original operations continued into the Medieval period in Western Europe, making a total of 1300 years without any original operations.

Traditional histories of surgery do not account for the absence of original operations during this lengthy period of time, as they concentrate on the actual operations performed by the Byzantines, Arabians and early Medieval surgeons, without noting they had all originated in antiquity.

These facts may have been described in this book for the first time. This will be further elaborated in subsequent chapters.

3. How Greek philosophy of surgery reached Western Europe.

In earlier chapters, Hippocrates' framework for the practice of surgery has been described, and it served a valuable purpose until the actual causes of diseases were discovered. It is also common knowledge, that following several translations, his manuscripts along with those of Aristotle and Galen, reached Western Europe in the early Middle Ages. How they finally got there is a complex tale and is presented here in chronological order. What stands out is the diligence and dedication of the scholars of successive empires and countries who translated the works of the Ancient Greeks during their years of power.

2nd Century BC. Hippocrates and the first translations.

The Greeks produced an intellectual and philosophical revolution that was coupled to Hippocrates' (460–370 BC)[21] theory and practice of medicine and surgery. The first translations of his manuscripts took place after they had been transferred to the Museum and Library in Alexandria in Egypt founded in about 285 BC having been modelled on Plato's Academy in Athens. From Alexandria, his manuscripts were transferred to Syria and translated into Syriac, the language of the ancient Assyrians and Persians. These translations were studied by Syrian physicians for centuries.

c387 BC. The foundation of Plato's Academy.

Plato (c428–347 BC) founded his Academy in Athens in c387 BC, followed by Aristotle (384–322 BC) who founded the Lyceum, also in Athens in 335 BC. Copies of their manuscripts were transferred to Alexandria in Egypt at some point before Athens was sacked in 87 BC by the Romans, that also resulted in the closure of the Academy and Lyceum.

In the Christian era, during the 3rd century, independent monasteries were being founded in Byzantium, where monks made copies of Hippocrates' and Galen's treatises. As time passed, some of these remained stored and forgotten in the monastic 'scriptoria', where they remained for over a thousand years before being rediscovered.

431 AD. The exile of Nestorius from Byzantium.

The Roman Emperor Theodosius II of Byzantium, exiled Nestorius,[22] (401-450) the Patriarch of Constantinople, for heresy in 431. Nestorius fled to Egypt with many of his followers, while others fled to Edessa in Mesopotamia. Amongst the migrants to Edessa were scholars who started to translate the Greek works of Galen (130–c200) into Syriac. Galen's writings included lengthy commentaries on the works of Herophilos[23] (335–280 BC) and Erasistratus[24] (c304–c250 BC), both famous anatomists, whose works were preserved for posterity by Galen as their original manuscripts were lost.

Nearly sixty years later in 489, another Byzantine army was once more pursuing the Nestorians in Edessa. They fled again and found refuge in the city of Gundê-Shãpūr in Persia.[25] Once settled, they not only continued to translate the Ancient Greek texts into Syriac, but also modelled their school on Greek lines. This Greek school in Gundê-Shãpūr was later claimed to be the birthplace of Arabic medicine.

529. Destruction of the Library in Alexandria in Egypt

As Byzantine intolerance of any deviation from Orthodox Christianity grew, Justinian the First (482-565) in his drive for religious uniformity banished what he called the heathen philosophers from the schools of Athens and Alexandria in Egypt in 529. Many of these scholars now followed the earlier migrations of the Nestorians[26] to Persia. Meanwhile, 'fanatical' Christians destroyed much of the Library in Alexandria in their attempt to 'root out heresy' from philosophical manuscripts.

622. John the Grammarian and Aaron the Presbyter.

The most important translations of the Greek manuscripts into Syriac were accomplished in Persia by John the Grammarian and Aaron the Presbyter about 622. They compiled thirty books in Syriac, called the *Pandect's of Aaron,* which were the last translations of Greek into Syriac.[27]

632 to 732. The Arab conquests.

Muslim armies conquered Arabia, followed by Syria, Palestine, Egypt, North Africa and Spain. Their advance in the West was finally halted at the Battle of Poitiers in France in 732. In the East, they conquered Persia and lands as far as China where they defeated a Chinese army. Chinese medical texts were sought in the 13th century but there was little written about surgery.[28]

636. The Academy at Gundê-Shäpūr

In 636, Gundê-Shäpūr was conquered by a Muslim army. The history of Gundê-Shäpūr as a great centre of learning is controversial. Be that as it may, it does not alter the overall thread of events presented here, for in about 683, a Syrian Jew called Maserjawaihi[29] had started to translate the Syriac manuscripts of Hippocrates and Galen into Arabic. This was the first definitive attempt to translate the medicine and surgery of the Greeks into the language of the Muslims. Meanwhile, the Nestorians, following the subjugation of Persia by an Arab army, were unharmed because of their monotheistic beliefs and in time became 'Arabised', taking Arab names and speaking Arabic as their first language. Their scholarship stood them in good stead, for when the Caliphs settled in Baghdad and turned their attention to historic and intellectual pursuits, they employed the Nestorians to translate the Ancient Greek documents from Greek or Syriac, into Arabic. Copies of these documents were also transferred to the Umayyad Caliphate in Spain where they were much later translated into Latin[30] after the fall of Toledo to the Christians in 1084–5.

c640. Paul of Aegina the last Byzantine surgeon.

The last of the Greek Byzantine surgeons was Paul of Aegina (615–690),[31] who lived at the time of the Muslim conquests and travelled among the Arabs where he was much in demand as an obstetrician. He copied from Galen and other Greek writers and his great treatise the *Epitome* became the standard text of the time. The *Epitome* was of particular interest to Muslim physicians and much later to the university scholars of Western Europe during the Middle Ages. It had been translated into Arabic by Albucasis,[32] al-Zahrāwi, Abu al-Qāsim.

762. Baghdad becomes the capital of the Eastern Caliphate.

In the 7th century, the works of Aristotle, Hippocrates and Galen were discovered in the Library in Alexandria and many were later transferred to Baghdad when it became the Caliph's capital city in 762. Muslim scholars accepted much of Aristotle's teachings, considering him a monotheist,[33] and spread his and Plato's philosophy throughout the Caliphates. They revived the School of Alexandria which once again flourished owing to the work of John the Grammarian[34] whose Arabic name was Yahyā al-Nahwī. The curriculum he laid down in Alexandria at that time consisted of sixteen texts by Galen that formed the basis of his lectures in Arabic.

The Muslims inherited 'the sciences' from the Greeks. Then, with their translations and their own interpretations of the Greek documents, they made Greek philosophy, medicine and surgery their own. They did this by aligning all the Greek treatises now in Arabic to their own way of thinking.[35] This was during the golden age in Baghdad between 750 and 850, a period of great intellectual curiosity. Arabic independent medical literature began in the 9th century and despite making significant advances in medicine and pharmacology, they were unable to advance surgery and undertook no original operations for reasons already described.

Turning West in 665, the systematic conquest of North Africa by Muslim armies was complete and in 670 the city of Kairawan was founded to the south of modern Tunis. It was from Kairawan that the Arabs initially governed their new territory in Spain during the next century and named it Al-Andalus. A University was founded in Cordova, in what became the Western Islamic Caliphate. Interestingly, Scholars from Europe began to arrive to take up 'Saracenic Studies' and took their learning back to Europe. The library in Cordova was estimated to contain 225,000 volumes or manuscripts. This included the works of Hippocrates, Plato, Aristotle and Galen translated into Arabic. At this time, Baghdad in the East and Cordova in the West had a regular interchange of knowledge, including philosophy, astronomy, mathematics as well as medicine and surgery. The intellectual curiosity of the Arabs had brought them the treasure houses of Persia and Egypt, including the manuscripts from the Museum and Library of Alexandria.

8th Century. The Nestorians in Baghdad.

Between the 8th and 11th centuries, it is believed that twelve generations of the Bukhtishu family of Nestorians served the Caliphs of Baghdad as physicians and translators, having risen to great prominence following their migration from Mesopotamia. One Nestorian, Hunayan ibn Ishāque,[36]who worked during the Golden Age of the Abbasid Califate in Baghdad and had mastered four languages, Arabic, Syriac, Greek and Persian and was known as the 'Sheikh of Translators'. His translations were well read and distributed throughout the Arab world. During his lifetime, he translated 116 works into Arabic and also produced 36 books of his own, 21 of which covered the field of medicine and included his *Ten Treatises on Ophthalmology*. He was also placed in charge of the famous 'House of Wisdom', the 'Bayt al Hikmah' in Baghdad by the 7th Abbasid Caliph, al-Ma'mūn.[37] He continued his work with *An Introduction to Medicine* and the translation of Galen's Commentaries and many other books into Arabic.

The story of Gundê-Shāpūr as a great centre of learning has since been challenged. It seems possible that the Nestorian scholars who migrated from there to Baghdad may have invented an increasingly illustrious history of it as a great centre of learning, in order to magnify their own importance to the Caliph in Baghdad. However, it was the Nestorians from Gundê-Shāpūr who were among the great scholars who continued to translate the Greek and Syriac versions of the Greeks into Arabic and align their philosophy with Islam.

850. The Indian Connection and Sushruta's Compendium.

In about 850, Sushruta's Compendium, an ancient Sanskrit text on medicine and surgery, was translated into Persian and then into Arabic as the *Kitab Shar Shun al Hindi* by Ali ibn Rabban al-Tabarī (f 850).[38] The surgical works of Sushruta were later translated into Latin in the early 1800s by Muller in Germany and in 1907 into English by Kaviraj Kunja lal Bhishagratna.[39]

These writings revealed and introduced Sushruta's plastic surgery and other operations to the West Europeans. There remains the open question of earlier contact concerning surgery between the Ancient Greeks and Indians. There is evidence that there were schools of medicine in India,[40] that did not have a fixed base and walked from town to town.

The operation to excise bladder stones was known to both Hippocrates in Greece and Sushruta in India. During the times of the Caliphates, couching of cataracts was also introduced from India and widely copied and practised by surgeons in Arabia and later in Europe.[41]

9th Century. Baghdad. The Caliph al Ma'mūn.

There was another reason that the Caliph al Ma'mūn (786–833) wished to study the translations of the Greek works. He was interested in a sect called the Mu'tazilites[42] who believed faith could be supported by 'radiocination', a process of thought accompanied by structured discussion. al Ma'mūn commissioned further translations of philosophical Greek documents to better clarify this matter.

9th century. Hunayn ibn-Ishāque. ue. *The Isogoge.*

In the 9th century, Hunayan ibn Ishāque. (809–873) whom we have already met was later known as Johannitus in the Latin West. The most important of his translations into Arabic was the *'Isogoge'*. This was translated into Latin by

Marcus of Toledo as *Liber Introductionis Medicina,* following the fall of Toledo to a Christian army in 1084. This was a systematic review of Galen's medicine that ultimately reached Latin Europe and in the later Middle Ages became an introductory medical textbook. This was the first example of an Arabic text being translated into Latin.[43]

9th Century. Baghdad. Abu Yusef al-Kindi.

In the 9th century, with the Caliphs in Baghdad, a Golden Age of scholarship followed. This was when 'The House of Wisdom' was established and among the scholars was Abu Yusef al-Kindi[44] (d after 873), known in the West as Alkindus. He translated Plato's philosophy into Arabic and revised the previous Arabic translation of Aristotle, setting the standard for later Arabic writers on philosophy by aligning these texts to the teachings of Islam.

He also studied optics and pharmacology.[45] In this period, some of the original operations by the Egyptians, Greeks and Hindus of India began to be copied and practiced as shown in the Box 9.1.

c900. Rhazes (841-962). Rāzi, Abu Bakr Muhammad ibn Zakaiyya. *The Golden Age in Baghdad.*

Rhazes' classification of infectious diseases replaced and updated those of Galen. He came to influence Albucasis (936–1013)[46] and Avicenna (c980–1037).

At this time, the Nestorians continued to translate the Syriac treatises into Arabic and at the same time to create a fusion of the Greek with the Islamic element of Arabic medicine, so as to align the original Greek philosophy with the teachings of Islam. This became unexpectedly useful to the advancement of science in Western Europe a few centuries later, as has already been noted.

In Baghdad, progress was made in literature, philosophy, astronomy and mathematics as well as medicine. As a result of their translations, Greek medicine as well as some elements of other medical traditions, were transformed, assimilated, adapted and finally adopted in the truest sense of the word into and as an integral part of Islamic culture.[47]

The Eastern Abbasid Caliphate in Baghdad was now at the zenith of the classical period of Arabian medicine. Rhazes (c849–926) was selected by the

Caliph for his medical skills to be in charge of the hospital in Baghdad. He is thought to be the most original of the Arabic commentators and translated both Hippocrates' and Galen's treatises into Arabic and followed their methods and ideas.[48]

One of Rhazes most interesting comments on these documents was that, 'When Galen and Aristotle are unanimous in the expression of an opinion, there lies the absolute truth, but when they are at variance it is hard to decide and we should (then) arrive at the proper course (decision) by ratiocination'. This format for deciding the truth was to continue for nearly a thousand years and became a characteristic of the Arabian schools in Spain where 'dialectic tournaments' among students took place to reach the truth of an opinion.

The truth was then arrived at by thinking about the problem and by structured argument.[49] This method of eliciting the 'truth' in any disagreement was also commonly practiced in Cordoba and Toledo in Muslim Spain and later taken up in the new Western European universities. The High Scholastics of Medieval Europe continued this practice of disputation to settle arguments by using the rules that had first been laid down by the early Greek philosophers.

Rhazes' most important works were translated into Latin as *Liber Almansorum and Continens* and was used as a textbook throughout the late Middle Ages. A copy in thirteen volumes in Latin reached the University of Paris in 1395. This textbook by Rhazes[50] was the longest and largest written before 1500 in the Eastern Caliphate. He improved clinical diagnosis and was the first to differentiate smallpox from measles. He produced a treatise on 'Examining the Physician' with quotations from Hippocrates and Galen. He also defined questions to ask students when assessing their suitability to become physicians.

His contemporaries nicknamed him the 'experienced' and he followed both Hippocrates and Galen in their methods and ideas. Rhazes in the Eastern Caliphate and Albucasis in the Western Caliphate were the leaders in abstract thought and were studied in the Middle Ages in Europe. His medical output was produced in ten volumes in *al-Kitabu-l-Mansuri, that* was translated into Latin by Gerard of Cremona in the 11th century. Rhazes book on anatomy and physiology is thought to be taken chiefly from Hippocrates and Galen. There was further refinement over the next 250 years and his book was translated into Latin as, *Liber de Medicina ad Almansorum* and formed part of the medical curriculum in the universities of Europe in the 16th century.

c1025. Avicenna. ibn Sīna, *and the Canon based on Galen's manuscripts.*

The most famous physician and philosopher of the Eastern Caliphate was Avicenna (980–1037), whose Arabic name was Ibn Sīna, .[51] He quoted Galen's dictum that surgery was inferior to medicine, an idea that slowly gained ground and may well have been cause of the Edict of Tours of 1163, as being too inferior a practice for physicians who were all university graduates at that time. He wrote many books and presented the doctrines of Hippocrates and Galen as modified by Aristotle, but with an Arabic interpretation. His greatest work was the *Canon* based on Galen's medical and surgical writings that he aligned to the teachings of Islam. It was soon translated from Arabic into Latin after the fall of Toledo, where this new source of Latin translations compared favourably to those of Constantine the African[52] c1060, who had also translated Galen's treatises into Latin at Monte Cassino in Italy. All these translations into Latin contained Arabist interpretations and both ultimately reached Western Europe.

Avicenna (c980–1037) declared, 'Medicine is a science from which one learns the states of the human body with respect to what is healthy and what is not, in order to preserve the good health when it exists and restore it when it is lacking'. He described the division between diseases that only affected one part of the body from those not specific to any part of the body. In the first came wounds and injuries and in the second category, he presented the symptoms and treatments. These were then divided into fevers, pustules, ulcers, swellings, leprosy, smallpox, wounds that had progressed to generalised sepsis, obesity, fractures and dislocations, poisons and animal and insect bites. He listed twenty-three types of fever and systematised and synthesised the Greek medical literature. His *Canon* came to dominate medicine in the Islamic world and then Medieval Europe, where it was used as a medical textbook for several centuries.[53]

Avicenna's writings were of the greatest interest to the Christian Scholastics. He presents the works of Hippocrates and Galen and aligned them with the teachings of Islam. 'Just as St Thomas Aquinas (1224-1274), who was educated at the Arabist centre at Naples two centuries later, aligned them with the Church'.[54] This train of thought eventually led to the beginning of science in Western Europe as described earlier in this chapter and is elaborated in Chapter 11.

The Canon was the final compilation of Graeco-Arabic medicine and formed half the medical curriculum of European Universities from the late 1400s to about 1650. This was the book that most excited the 'scholastics' in the universities of Europe. For they especially admired the most obscure passages which they considered so complex and brilliant that when it was beyond their comprehension, they believed that it was therefore sublime.[55]

c1060. Italy. Constantinus Africanus. Translation of Ancient Greek and Arabic medical texts into Latin.

Constantine, the African (c1020–1087), was a Christian monk. Born in Carthage in North Africa, he later travelled widely in Syria, India, Ethiopia, Persia and Egypt. He studied at the famous medical school in Salerno in Southern Italy and then entered the Monastery at Monte Cassino, founded in 529. There he translated into Latin the works of Hippocrates and Galen from the Greek. He also translated thirty-seven books from Arabic into Latin, including two treatises by Isaac Judaeus (850-941),[56] who was considered the greatest physician of the Western Caliphate in Al-Andalus. He also translated the works of the Arab physicians Razes and Avicenna. Constantine was one of the first scholars to bring these texts to Western Europe.

1085. Toledo in Spain. A city famous as a seat for translations from Greek to Arabic and later from Arabic to Latin.

After the fall of Toledo to a Christian army in 1085, Gerard of Cremona[57] an Italian scholar, was sent by the Holy Roman Emperor to translate the works of Avicenna from Arabic into Latin. In Toledo Gerard learnt perfect Arabic having been taught by Ibn Ghalib, a native Christian writer. Gerard was the first European to delight in and translate the subtlety of the Arabised Greek medicine and surgery. In all, he translated seventy Arabic works including Avicenna's *Canon* into Latin. His translations spread quickly throughout Western Europe during the 12th century and the university scholars who most admired these Arabist interpretations became known as 'Scholastics'.[58] Avicenna's Canon was so appreciated that it made up half of the medical curriculum in European Universities until the end of the 15th century. Unfortunately, it was he who drew attention to Galen's opinion that surgery was a 'minor' branch of medicine with unfortunate consequences. This was taken up by the scholars in medieval Europe, who were Arabists and considered the human body unclean, so surgery that inevitably involved contact with blood and pus fell into this category. This led to the Edict of Tours in 1163.

Meanwhile, the Italian and later the European 'Scholastic' professors were 'ecstatic' for they considered the *Canon* to be the 'foundations apparently immutable of knowledge'. They believed that Galen's writings could not be surpassed and were literally the final revelation of knowledge as far as anatomy, medicine and surgery were concerned. Avicenna's complex reasoning further appealed to the Scholastics because they were able to find the utmost subtlety in passages of his interpretation of Galen's treatises. Anything that was obscure or even unintelligible they considered the most learned and sublime of mystical writing, a concept that understandably most modern minds have difficulty grasping, because if it was unintelligible, it may merely have been an inaccurate translation, but that is not how the scholastics thought. Despite or because of this, the influence of the *Canon* in Western Europe continued to the end of the Middle Ages.

12th century. Averroes., I ibn-Ruschd, Abū al-Walīd and the end of liberal thought in Spain.

Change was now taking place in Muslim Spain. Averroes (1126–1198)[59] was born in Cordoba in the Western Caliphate and studied philosophy, law and medicine. He particularly admired the works of Aristotle and was a free thinker and this cast doubt on his religious adherence. This resulted in his dismissal from office as the governor of Seville. He died in prison in Morocco. The previous liberal culture of learning now passed away and a return to orthodox Islam took place from and after 1195. This was rapidly followed by the disappearance of speculative thought among Arab scholars.

1204. The Fourth Crusade and the sack of Constantinople.

A catastrophe occurred when the Christian army of the 4th Crusade sacked Constantinople[60] in 1204 while on their way to the Holy Land. This caused great instability in Byzantium and not only Constantinople but also many monasteries were ransacked. It was in this uncertain period that the monks rediscovered their ancient copies of Greek texts by Hippocrates, Aristotle and Galen that had lain in their scriptoria for a thousand years, albeit ignored and sometimes overwritten. These they sent to Italy, where they were translated into Latin and because they came directly from Byzantium, they naturally contained no Arabic commentaries or interpretations.

Many of these Greek manuscripts still exist and when they first reached the European Universities their contents dismayed the Scholastic professors, who loved the 'Arabist' or Islamic interpretations of Greek philosophy and medicine. The Scholastics were further challenged by a new revolution in thought that began to displace both the Scholastic and the 'Hellenistic' interpretations of Ancient Greek philosophy. This new revolution was the conception and subsequent development of science.

1235. The fall of Cordova.

The Western Caliphate's capital in Spain fell to the Christians in 1235 and less than 30 years later, the capital of the Eastern Caliphate in Baghdad was sacked by the Mongols in 1259. These cataclysmic events brought an end to Arabic translations and interpretations of the intellectual works of the Greeks.

In spite of this decline, the Arabist translation of Galen's book *Chirurgia Magna* was so influential in Europe that it was printed through 52 editions, the last being in 1622. The translator was Guy de Chauliac (d. 1368), a Frenchman and a 'Scholastic'[61] whose book also plagiarised Galen's treatise on anatomy. These translations of Razes' books remained in print even longer, the last edition being printed in 1781, giving a final boost of support to the High Scholastics.

The question of the distribution and availability in Europe of the Latin translations of Galen's most studied work, *Ars Medica,* the *Art of Medicine*, was undertaken by Dr Donald Campbell in 1926.[62] He recorded copies in 54 cities. The most important of these, in alphabetical order, were Cambridge, Copenhagen, Dresden, Edinburgh, Hamburg, London, Madrid, Munich, Montpellier, Oxford, Padua and Paris. This wide distribution confirms the continuing importance attached to Galen's writing. However, during the late Middle Ages, the omniscience of the Ancient Greeks began to decline, but despite this, the teachings of the 'Scholastic and Hellenistic' professors in the universities remained dominant.

Meanwhile, outside the universities, doubts concerning Galen's infallibility as the final and enduring authority on practical surgery were beginning to take hold. The turning point came during the never-ending European wars when discussion of how to treat gunshot wounds arose. Unsurprisingly there was no help to be found in the writings of Hippocrates or Galen. For 'wounds (were now) proving better teachers of surgery than any faculty of medicine'. This now had a ring of truth to it, especially as surgery had been deleted from the university curriculum following the Edict of Tours of 1163.[63]

Gradually, it was being realised that under the Scholastic professors, medicine was no longer a going concern. It had become a static, doctrinal and unchangeable dogma, analogous to a religion. Changing their approach to medicine was not then possible because there was nothing at that time to replace the established Greek theory of disease propounded by Hippocrates. This resulted in his theory of medical practice remaining the only intellectual framework within which medicine and surgery could continue to be practised.

c1246. Ayyubid Sultanate. Ibn al-Nafīs. *Cairo. Discovery of the pulmonary circulation.*

A significant anatomical discovery occurred during the Ayyubid Sultanate. This was the discovery of the pulmonary circulation by Ibn al-Nafīs (1213–1288), a Syrian physician who spent most of his life at the Museum in Cairo. He asserted correctly that the blood in the right ventricle of the heart must reach the left ventricle by way of the lungs alone and denied that there was any direct connection between the ventricles.[64] This was a significant advance on Galen's anatomy. Ibn al-Nafīs' work was unusual as Islamic writings on anatomy were conservative and otherwise deviated little from their Greek models, at a time when human dissection was forbidden.

The discovery of the circulation of the blood through the body, had to wait another four hundred years, until Dr William Harvey[65] (1588–1658) performed his meticulous research and published, *De Motu Cordis* and *De Circulatione Sanguinis* in 1628 in Frankfurt in Latin. He correctly described the function of both ventricles and the role of the arteries and veins in delivering and receiving blood from the organs. The presence of capillaries was discovered soon afterwards.

In anatomy, it was Galen's meticulous dissections of macaques that reached Western Europe and became the anatomy textbook used for centuries. For Ibn al-Nafīs' anatomical studies of the heart and his study of the eyes were exceptional discoveries as noted by Hunayn ibn Ishāq. (d 873 or 877) in his *Ten Treatises on the eye.* [66]

1289. The University of Montpellier.

In Montpellier, the 'Scholastic' interpretation of the Greek writings remained dominant. Copies of Hippocrates' works were transferred to the University of Montpellier, one of the first European Universities founded in 1289. There, the Latin 'Arabist' translations of Constantine the African[67] (102–1087) from Monte Cassino in Italy and of Gerard of Cremona (1114–1187) from Toledo were also gathered. Constantine, in addition to the medical works, also introduced Arabic numerals and lengthy Arabic pharmacopoeias. The Arabic numerals were the foundation for developing modern mathematics and the pharmacopoeias were extensively used in Western Europe during the Middle Ages.

The transfer of Ancient Greek surgery to Western Europe has now been outlined. Its impact on Surgery during the Middle Ages is further elaborated in Chapter 12.

References:

1. Chapter 2. 1,700 BC. Incision of abscesses.
2. Ibid. c425 BC. Excision of bladder stones.
3. Ibid. c425 BC. Venesection.
4. Ibid. c1,700 BC. Reduction of dislocations.
5. Ibid. c1,700 BC. Setting of fractures.
6. Ibid. c30 AD. Tonsillectomy.
7. Ibid. c200 BC. Couching of cataracts.
8. Ibid. c2,500 BC. Circumcision.
9. Ibid. c10,000 BC. Trephination of the skull.
10. Ibid. c30 AD. Inguinal hernia repair.
11. Ibid. c425 BC. Haemorrhoidectomy.
12. Ibid. c30 AD. Amputation
13. Ibid. c425 BC. Fistula-in-ano.

14. Ibid. c30 AD. Hydrocele.
15. Ibid. c30 AD. Closure of abdomen.
16. Ibid. c170 AD. Tracheostomy.
17. *Medieval Islamic Medicine.* By Peter Pormann & Emilie Savage-Smith. The New Edinburgh Islamic Surveys. Edinburgh University Press Ltd. Reprinted 2010. ISBN. 978 0 7486 2067 8.
18. Acculturation. *Medieval Islamic Medicine.* By Peter E. Pormann & Emilie Savage-Smith. The New Edinburgh Islamic Surveys. Edinburgh University Press Ltd. Reprinted 2010, p 12–15.
19. p 36–37.
20. *The Beginnings of Western Science. The European Scientific Tradition in Philosophical, Religious and Institutional Context, 600 BC to AD 1450.* By David C. Lindberg. The University of Chicago Press. 1992, p 240–244.
21. Chapter 2, c425 BC. Hippocrates.
22. *Ditto. Nestorius.431 AD*
23. *Arabian Medicine. Vol. 1.* By Dr Donald Campbell. Keegan Paul, Trench and Trubner. London, 1926. Herophilos.
24. Chapter 2, c260 BC, Erasistratus.
25. *Arabian Medicine. Vol. 1.* By Dr Donald Campbell. Keegan Paul, Trench and Trubner. London, 1926, p 46, 48, 60. Gundê-Shãpūr.
26. *Medieval Islamic Medicine.* By Peter E. Pormann and Emile Savage-Smith. The new Edinburgh Islamic Surveys. Edinburgh University Press. 2010. p 20, 21, 35. The Nestorians as translators.
27. *Arabian Medicine and its Influence on the Middle Ages. Vol. 1.* By Dr Donald Campbell. Keegan Paul, Trench and Trubner. London, 1926, p 47. The Pandects.
28. *Medieval Islamic Medicine*. By Peter Pormann & Emilie Savage-Smith. The New Edinburg Islamic Surveys. Edinburgh University Press Ltd., 2010, Surgery in China, p 21–23.
29. *Arabian Medicine and its Influence on the Middle Ages. Vol 1.* By Dr Donald Campbell. Keegan Paul, Trench and Trubner. London, 1926, p 47. Maserjawaihi.
30. *Medieval Islamic Medicine.* By Peter E. Pormann and Emile Savage-Smith. The New Edinburgh Islamic Surveys. Edinburgh University Press. 2010, p 164, Toledo.

31. *Arabian Medicine. Vol.1.* Dr Donald Campbell. 1926. Keegan Paul, Trench and Trubner. London, 1926, p 11–12. Paul of Aegina.
32. *Arabian Medicine. Vol. II.* Dr Donald Campbell. Keegan Paul, Trench and Trubner. London. 1926, p 85–87. Abucasis
33. *Aristotle.* By A.E. Taylor. Dover Publication Inc., N.Y. ISBN 10: 0-486-20280-1. First published in 1919. Reprinted 1955, p 86–87. Monotheism.
34. *Arabian Medicine.* Vol. 1. Dr Donald Campbell. 1926. Keegan Paul, Trench and Trubner. London, Vol. 1. 1926, p 47, 50. John the Grammarian.
35. *Arabian Medicine.* Vol. 1. Dr Donald Campbell. Keegan Paul, Trench and Trubner. London. 1926, p 79. Dialectical subtlety.
36. *Medieval Islamic Medicine.* Peter E. Pormann and Emile Savage-Smith. The New Edinburgh Islamic Surveys. Edinburgh University Press. 2010, p 25-33. Hunayan ibn Ishaque.
37. Wikipedia. The Caliph al Ma'mun.
38. *Medieval Islamic Medicine.* Peter E. Pormann and Emile Savage-Smith. The New Edinburgh Islamic Surveys. Edinburgh University Press. 2010, p 35, 36, 37. Ali ibn Rabban al-Tabarî
39. *An English Translation of the Sushruta Samhita, based on original Sanskrit text.* By Kavirag Kunja Lal Bhishagratna. Published by S'L' Bhaduri. Calcutta, 1916. Reprinted by Nabu Public Domain Reprints 2019.
40. *A History of Medicine. Vol, II. Early Greek, Hindu and Persian Medicine.* By Henry E. Sigerist. Oxford University Press. 1961, p 185. Surgical schools in India.
41. *Medieval Islamic Medicine.* By Peter E. Pormann and Emlie Savage-Smith. The New Edinburgh Islamic Surveys. Editor Carole Hillenbrand. Edinburgh University Press. Reprinted 2010, p 127–128. Couching of cataracts.
42. Wikipedia. The Mut'tazalites.
43. *Arabian Medicine. Vol. 1.* Dr Donald Campbell. Keegan Paul, Trench and Trubner. 1926, p 137–138. First Arabic texts translated into Latin.
44. *Arabian Medicine. Vol. 1.* Dr Donald Campbell. Keegan Paul, Trench and Trubner. 1926, p 63, 64. Al-Kindi.

45. *Medieval Islamic Medicine* by P.E. Pormann & E. Savage-Smith. Edinburgh University Press, 2010, p 54. Pharmacology.
46. *Arabian Medicine. Vol. I.* Dr Donald Campbell. Keegan Paul, Trench and Trubner. London. 1926, p 85–87. Abucasis.
47. *Medieval Islamic Medicine.* By P.E. Pormann & E. Savage-Smith. Edinburgh University Press, 2010, p 37. Assimilation into Islamic culture.
48. *Arabian Medicine and its Influence on the Middle Ages. Vol. 1.* By Dr Donald Campbell. London. Kegan Paul, Trench, Trubner & Co., Ltd. 1926, p 70, 71. Al-Razi's translations.
49. *Arabian Medicine and its Influence on the Middle Ages. Vol. 1.* By Dr Donald Campbell. London. Kegan Paul, Trench, Trubner & Co., p 72. Ratiocination.
50. *Ibid. 68. Liber ad Almansorum and Continens.*
51. *Ibid. 129. Surgery an inferior branch of medicine.*
52. *Ibid. 122. Constantine the African.*
53. *Ibid. 79. The Cannon of Avicenna. And, The Canon of Medicine.*
54. St Thomas Aquinas. Dr Donald Campbell. Keegan Paul, Trench and Trubner. London. 1926.
55. The Scholastics. Arabian Medicine. Dr Donald Campbell. Keegan Paul, Trench and Trubner. London. 1926, P. 154
56. *Ibid. 73. Isaac Judaeus.*
57. *Ibid. 124. Gerard of Cremona.*
58. *Ibid. 79. The Scholastics.*
59. *Ibid. 92–96. Averroes.*
60. *The Sack of Constantinople by the Fourth Crusade.* Wikipedia.
61. *The beginnings of Western Science. The European Scientific Tradition in Philosophical, Religious, and Institutional Context, 600 BC to AD 1450.* The University of Chicago Press, 1992, p 341, 343. Guy de Chauliac.
62. *Arabian Medicine. Vol. 1.* Dr Donald Campbell. Keegan Paul, Trench and Trubner. London. 1926, p 19–25. Ars Medica in the libraries of Europe.
63. Chapter *2.* 1163. The Edict of Tours.

64. *Medieval Islamic Medicine*. Peter E. Pormann & Emily Savage Smith. Edinburgh University Press. 2010. ISBN 988 0 7486 2066 1, p 46, 47. The lesser circulation through the lungs.
65. *De Motu Cordis et de Circulatione Sanguinis. The Anatomical Exercises by William Harvey*. Edited by Geoffrey Keynes. Dover Publications Inc, New York. The first English text of 1653, reprinted 1995. And Chapter 2. 1628. Dr William Harvey
66. *Arabian Medicine. Vol. 1.* Dr Donald Campbell. 1926. Keegan Paul, Trench and Trubner. London, Vol. 1. 1926, p 49. Hunayan ibn Ishaque. Ten Treatises on the Eye.
67. *Ibid. 130. Constantine the African.*

Chapter 10: Fourth Period

1085 to 1845. Surgery in Medieval Western Europe and the USA

Original Operations in Late Medieval and Early Modern Western Europe and the Early Modern United States of America with Subsequent Developments

The oldest university in Italy was Bologna, founded in 1088. Oxford University grew informally from 1096 and was recognised as a university by 1167. Cambridge Universitywas founded in 1231, the Sorbonne in Paris in 1258 and Montpellier in 1289. Many more followed. The universities of Medieval Europe were receiving and studying the ancient writings of the Greeks, now translated from Arabic into Latin, the language of medieval educated Europeans. Later the works of Hippocrates and Galen were translated into the vernacular languages of Europe.

Students from all over Europe attended the Italian universities including John of Arderne (1307-1380) and William Harvey (1578-1657). The Greek subjects being taught included philosophy, astronomy, mathematics, medicine and surgery.

Handwritten manuscripts of English translations of John of Arderns's Latin writings were produced in the 1400s and became available to surgeons in England.

Technological innovations introduced to Europe that had an impact on surgery, included gunpowder from China, about which we will learn more. Also, many Arabic words were absorbed into the European languages, such as alchemy (chemistry), algebra, sugar, camphor and cotton.

Reference:

Fifteenth century Manuscript of John of Arderne Medical Treatises in English. Glasgow University Library, Special Collections Department. 2006.

1163. France. The Edict of Tours.

The practice of surgery changed dramatically in Western Europe when in 1163 Pope Alexander the Third at the Council of Tours pronounced an Edict, 'Ecclesia Abhorret a Sanguine'. This is loosely translated as the, 'Church is opposed to the shedding of blood by the clergy'. Widely interpreted by the clerics to mean that physicians who were all university educated and members of the clergy were now forbidden to spill blood by practicing surgery.

There were claims that the Pope never made any such pronouncement. However, Canon 8 of the Edict of Tours prohibited clerics from involving themselves in studies of a physical nature. The pope had declared that anyone undertaking such studies, 'Must be in league with the Devil'. The physicians, knowing perfectly well that surgery was a physical occupation, decided that they should, or was it could, now abandon surgery and proceeded to do so.[1]

From that time, the practice of surgery could not to be delegated and was completely dissociated from the practice of medicine. Professor Clifford T. Allbutt (1836–1925), Regius Professor of Physic at Cambridge University during a lecture in 1904, on the '*Historical Relations of Medicine and Surgery*', at St Louis in the USA, declared, "It was as though Medicine had lopped off its right arm by the expulsion of surgery from the liberal arts when this pernicious bisection of medicine was made." He continued, "Surgery, hated and avoided by Medical Faculties, scorned in clerical and feudal circles, began (to be practised) in the hands of lowly and uneducated men."

These were the barbers, shavers and haircutters who before the edict had been delegated by the clergy to preform minor surgical procedures such as venesection and lancing of abscesses and were now by default in charge of all the practice of surgery having been abandoned to fend for themselves.[2]

This dissociation had a devastating effect on the practice of surgery that was as 'profound as the situation was illogical'. For surgery had always been the active arm of medicine and in the times of the Ancient Egyptians was more advanced than medicine, the latter then being dominated by magic and incantations, while surgery was and always has been a practical craft. Forbidden entry to the universities on account of both their class and lack of education, the barbers over a long period of time began to organise themselves.

As Europe emerged from the dark ages, surgery after the 'Edict of Tours' was primitive and what little took place were the simplest procedures. Many surgeons then learned their craft in the hard school of war. But without proper guidance, they were in danger of compounding the errors of the past.[3]

Gradually, over a period of 700 years, the barber surgeons and later surgeons progressed on an entirely separate pathway from the physicians who were university trained. Through their own endeavour surgeons developed collegiate institutions, starting with guilds. Then they brought in apprenticeships and over the centuries were involved in what were to become teaching hospitals. In more modern times, they undertook and set examinations, and to this day, the Royal College of Surgeons, remain the authority in the United Kingdom to grant fellowships following success in a rigorous examination. When passed surgeons are qualified to practice surgery unsupervised.

References:

1. Constitutions of Clarendon: Council of Tours 1163. Conclarendon.blogpost.com
2. *The Historical Relations of Medicine and Surgery to the End of the Sixteenth Century.* T. Clifford Allbutt. Macmillan and Co, New York. 1905.
3. *The History of the Royal College of Surgeons of England.* By Zachary Cope. Published by Anthony Blond Ltd. 1959.

1252. France. Establishment of Surgical Guilds.

The first sign of surgeons organising themselves was when in 1252 a Guild of Barber-Surgeons was founded in Montpellier followed by Paris in 1260. In London, a Company of Barbers was formed in 1300 and later a Guild of surgeons, then in 1540 the Company of Barber-Surgeons was formed.

Reference:

The History of the Royal College of Surgeons of England. By Zachary Cope. Printed by Anthony Blond Ltd, London, 1959. Also, the website of the Royal College of Surgeons of England.

1258. Italy. Pus is not laudable.

Theodoric of Lucca (1205–1296), an Italian Dominican friar published a book, *Chirurgia* and in it disputed the teachings of Galen (c131–201 AD) and of the subsequent Arab authors concerning the nature of pus. It was generally believed that suppuration and the formation of pus was a normal process and necessary for wounds to heal. Theodoric disagreed and condemned the idea of 'laudable pus', when he wrote, 'as all modern surgeons profess, pus should be generated in wounds. No error can be greater than this. Such a practice is to hinder nature, to prolong the disease and prevent the consolidation of the wound'.[1]

Theodoric was right, but unfortunately before his time. He was not the first to be ignored in this matter, although he may have been aware that Galen when surgeon to the Gladiators in Pergamon from 158–61 AD had observed and written that some wounds healed without suppuration.[2] It was not until pathogenic bacteria and their role in sepsis was unravelled in the 19th century, that laudable pus was finally seen for what it was, an infection, a disease and not an intrinsic part of healing.

References:

1. *A History of Surgery.* By Harold Ellis. Published by Greenwich Medical Media Ltd. 2001.
2. *The Healing Hand.* By Guido Majno. Harvard University Press 1975, p 400. And Galen of Pergamon
3. by George Sarton. Pub. University of Kansas Press 1954. 183.

1300. England. From Surgical Guild to the Company of Surgeons of London.

During 1300, the first Guild of Surgeons was established in England. Surgery was still in total disarray following the Edict of Tours of 1163.[1] Strangely, it was unexpectedly helped in England by the Dissolution of the Monasteries that was ordered by King Henry the VIII and carried out between 1536 and 1539. One consequence of this was that many lay monks, not being priests or physicians, had a rudimentary knowledge of simple surgery and now had to seek employment elsewhere. This may have influenced Henry to unite the Barbers and Surgeons into a single Company of Barber-Surgeons that would also allow former monks to be admitted, this was by act of parliament in 1540. The creation of the Barber-Surgeons represented a slight improvement in the status of surgeons, although still inferior to the barbers, let alone the physicians.

It was in the 16th century that the works of Hippocrates and Galen were translated into English and therefore available to the generality of surgeons in England and Europe. Before that, we know that Chaucer, when writing *The Canterbury Tales,* towards the end of the fourteenth century, mentions in his Prologue that the Doctor was well-versed in the writings of Hippocrates, Galen, Rhazes and others and from this it can be assumed that the Pilgrims were familiar with these names. The Greek treatises of Hippocrates and Galen had been available in Latin since the 11th century, but sequestered in the Universities and unavailable to surgeons since the Edict of Tours of 1163. When the English translations of the Ancient Greek treatises were available, surgeons read about operations that had been practiced in antiquity and began to advance their own practise by copying them. This was further boosted when improvements in the understanding of anatomy followed Andreas Vesalius'[2] detailed dissections that were published in 1534.

It is interesting to realise, that it was the operations of the Ancients that were now being copied. Surgeons must have been encouraged that operations, such as hernia repair and surgery for fistula-in-ano, had been successfully carried out more than 1,500 years earlier. This proved that John of Arderne's fistula operation was not an original operation. There is only one example, among the original operations, that may have originated twice separately, but even that is extremely doubtful.[3]

Another advance was that members of the Barber-Surgeons Company were now encouraged to take prospective surgeons into a formal apprenticeship of seven years. At the same time, a Court of Examiners was elected by the surgeons to test the apprentices at the end of their term. If successful, they were entitled to practice in London as Freemen of the Barber-Surgeons Company, which controlled surgery in London for the next 200 years.[4]

As the power of the surgeons gradually increased, they eventually split from the Barbers to become the Company of Surgeons in 1745. The standard of surgery at that time is discussed in the next chapter.

References:

1. The Edict of Tours. This Chapter in 1163.
2. Vesalius. This Chapter in 1534.
3. John Hunter. This Chapter in 1785.
4. *The History of the Royal College of Surgeons of England.* By Zachary Cope. Pub. Anthony Blond Ltd. 1959.

1440. Germany. Printed books in Europe and the dissemination of knowledge.

The Renaissance in Europe spread rapidly from the south to the north as interest in the arts, science and medicine increased. The speed with which information was transmitted was revolutionised by the use of the printing press. In 1440 Johannes Gutenberg[1] (c1398–1468), a German in the Holy Roman Empire facilitated the rapid spread of knowledge through his printing. Within sixty years, more than twenty million books on many subjects had been produced.

It has been difficult to discover the first surgical text to have been printed on a Gutenberg type of press, Galen's *Tegni* otherwise known as *Ars Parva* was first published in Latin in Venice in 1496.[2]

The original inventors of printing were the Chinese during the Han Dynasty of 216 BC–220 AD. Their technique was to print on paper or cloth using texts carved on stone, later the templates were carved in wood.

References:

1. Wikipedia. Johannes Gutenberg.
2. Arabian Medicine and its Influence on the Middle Ages. Volume II. By Dr Donald Campbell. London, Kegan Paul, Trench, Trubner & Co. London. 1926. P.7.

1506. Italy. The foundation of pathological anatomy.

Antonio Benivieni (1448–1502), was a physician practising in Florence who founded the science of pathological anatomy. He insisted on the need for necropsy to reveal what he called the 'hidden causes' of diseases and was the first to ask, not what is disease, but 'where is it'. Benivieni's book, *De Abditis Causis Morborum* was published a year after his death. Among his pathological reports, he identified biliary calculi, abscesses of the mesentery, thrombosis of the mesenteric vessels, stenosis of the intestine, cardiac cases with polypus (blood clots), ruptured bowels, caries of the ribs that was so extensive that the heart was exposed and cancer of the stomach.[1] This was the first time that both physicians and surgeons began to learn what types of diseases could afflict the abdominal organs.

Giovanni Batista Morgagni (1682–1771), was an Italian anatomist who studied at Bologna and became Professor of Anatomy in Padua in Italy. In 1761, he also published a book concerning pathology in five volumes, *De Sedibus et Causis Morborum.* This was translated into French in 1765 and in English in 1769, under the title of the *Seats and Causes of Disease*. Morgagni described the anatomical changes in organs and tissues from his post-mortems on patients who had died of disease rather than being hanged as criminals. He established the fundamental principle that a large proportion of diseases are not vaguely dispersed throughout the body, but originate locally in specific organs and tissues.[2]

Benivieni and Morgagni gave practical substance to Avicenna (980-1037) who had been the first to divide diseases into those that affect only one part of the body and those not specific to any part of the body.[3]

References:

1. *The Historical Relations of Medicine and Surgery to the End of the Sixteenth Century.* An address delivered to the St Louis Congress in 1904 by T. Clifford Allbutt. St Louis 1904.
2. *A History of Surgery.* By Harold Ellis. Greenwich Medical Media Ltd. 2001, ISBN 1 84110 023 4.
3. Chapter 2. c1025. The Canon of Medicine.

1543. Italy. Anatomy becomes a modern science under Vesalius.

Galen (130–c200 AD) dissected many different species of animals because human dissections were forbidden. His dissections of Barbary macaques were meticulous, detailed and advanced for his time and were used by him as a proxy for human dissection. Subsequently, Galen's treatises were not added to or revised,[1] so knowledge of anatomy remained that of the macaques. Using ape anatomy was, to say the least, unhelpful as a proxy for humans, for not surprisingly important aspects of anatomy particularly in the differences between the skull and the pelvis were misleading. Despite this, Galen's anatomy became and remained the standard textbook for the next 1300 years. Andreas Vesalius[2] (1514–1564) was a Flemish anatomist who had read Galen's work and was fired with enthusiasm to revise human anatomical knowledge. He was appointed Professor of Surgery at Padua University at the age of 23 and there carried out his own meticulous dissections, that were then permitted on executed convicted criminals. These were public dissections that attracted wide audiences of surgeons and students from all over Europe who came to observe and learn.

Vesalius produced *De Humani Corporis Fabrica, The Structure of the Human Body,* published in 1543. He pointed out errors in Galen's work, showing for example that the human kidney is smooth while Galen had written that it was lobulated as in the pig. He also proved that there were no pores able to transport blood directly between the ventricles of the heart. Vesalius contributed a new thirst for knowledge and had the courage to challenge the errors of the ancients[2].

Between 1543–1846, the anatomical renaissance started by Vesalius began to make better sense of the connections between organs and tissues of the body. After general anaesthesia was introduced in 1846,[3] surgeons began to have enough knowledge to plan and carry out detailed elective operations. These were on patients with diseases that had previously been hidden inside the formerly unapproachable great cavities of the body.

King Henry VIII (1491–1547) granted permission that every year the bodies of four criminals who had been condemned to death were to be used for the teaching of anatomy. His daughter, Queen Elizabeththe First (1533–1603) granted a charter to Gonville and Caius College Cambridge in 1564, in which the Master and Fellows were allowed to take the bodies of two criminals who had been condemned to death and then executed in Cambridge. She decreed that the cadavers were to be given, 'Free of all charges, to be used for the purpose of dissection, with a view to the increase of knowledge of medicine and to benefit the health of her Majesty's lieges (subjects), without interference on the part of any of her officials'.[4] A telling aside possibly reflecting on the probity of the Royal servants in Tudor times.

References:

1. *Galen on Anatomical Procedures*. Translated by Charles Singer. Oxford University Press, 1956. Reprinted in 1999.
2. *Andreas Vesalius, the Reformer of Anatomy.* By James Moores Ball, Trieste 2017. ISBN 9880649026388.
3. Chapter 2. 1846. Ether.
4. *The Cambridge Illustrated History of Medicine.* Editor Roy Porter. Cambridge University Press, 1996.

1575. France. First transurethral prostatectomy.

This prostatectomy was the first original operation to be undertaken since Galen's original operation of suturing severed tendons and muscles, in about 180 AD, nearly 1400 years earlier.[1]

Ambroise Paré (1510–1590), is credited with the first transurethral prostatectomy, an original operation carried out on a patient in 1575. The operation was the first 'punch' partial prostatectomy. Paré used a hollow metal sound (catheter), that housed a sharp-edged hemispherical tip fastened to a wire that passed through the tube. The sound was introduced into the bladder and any part of an enlarged prostate that pressed against the blade would be pushed into the hollow space in the tube and amputated by withdrawing the wire. This pioneering work became the prototype of endoscopic prostatic surgery practiced today.[2]

Benign prostatic hyperplasia is a disease of middle aged and old men. In early antiquity, the average life span was considerably less than 40 years, so there would be few men affected by prostatism and regular catheterisation would be the usual treatment for those so afflicted.

With that in mind, the first recorded use of a catheter was in Ancient Egypt in about 3,000 BC, when straws or tubes of vegetable origin were used.[3] Celsus (c25 BC–c50 AD) records the use of catheters of various size and length in bronze.[4]

The first suprapubic approach to the bladder was by Dr Jean Amussat (1796–1856) in 1823. He was carrying out a suprapubic operation to remove a large bladder stone and incidentally found that there was also urinary retention caused by an enlarged middle lobe of the prostate which he excised.[5] This operation was carried out before the introduction of anaesthesia, it was not an original operation as it was already known that it was possible to operate on the prostate through a urethral approach.

In 1895, a simple prostatectomy for benign prostatic hypertrophy was carried out under general anaesthesia, through a suprapubic trans-vesical incision, by Dr Eugene Fuller (1858–1930) of New York. This operation was then popularised by Sir Peter Freyer (1851–1921) of St Peter's Hospital London.

In 1911, Dr Hugh H. Young[6] (1870–1945), an American surgeon and urologist, was appointed head of the Department of Urology at Johns Hopkins Hospital at the age of 27. He developed an instrument he called a 'punch' which updated Ambrose Paré's instrument. This was composed of a tube, that when incorporated into a rigid cystoscopy was used to carry out transurethral prostatectomies. Bleeding caused significant problems that were later solved by John Caulk (1881–1938) who introduced electric cautery to coagulate bleeding vessels. This became a standard instrument used during this operation.[7] He also carried out the first radical prostatectomy for cancer.[8]

Mr Terrence Millin (1903–1980) of London, in 1945, developed and popularised a retro-pubic approach to prostatectomy that avoided opening the bladder. It was still being routinely used in the UK into the 1970s[9] and thereafter was rapidly replaced by trans urethral prostatectomies. Not long afterwards, the new subspecialty of Urology was established in the UK. In modern times, radical robot assisted prostatectomy for cancer is discussed under the heading of Robotic Assisted Surgery.[9]

References:

1. *The Enlarged Prostate: A Brief History of its Surgical Treatment.* By Harry W Herr of the department of Urology, Sloan Kettering Cancer Centre, Cornell University Medical College, New York, onlinelibrary.wiley.com. BJU 2006 International.
2. *History of Surgery.* By Harold Ellis. Greenwich Medical Media Ltd. 2001.
3. *Celsus on Medicine. Loeb Classical Library. Volume II, Book 5.* With an English Translation by W.G. Spencer. Harvard University Press 1938. P. LX1
4. *History of Surgery.* By Harold Ellis. Greenwich Medical Media Ltd. 2001. p 120–123.
5. *Bailey and Love's Short Practice of Surgery.* By A.J. Harding Rains and H. David Ritchie. H.K. Lewis and Co. Ltd. 1977, p 1242.
6. *A History of Surgery.* By Harold Ellis. Greenwich Medical Media Ltd. 2001, ISBN 1 84110 023 4. p 123.
7. *The Royal College of Surgeons. Plarr's Lives of the Fellows.* Terrence Millin.
8. *The End of the Golden Age of General Surgery, 1870–2000.* By Nigel Keith Maybury. CreateSpace Independent Publishing Platform. North Charleston, South Carolina. p 29.
9. Chapter 14. 2000. Robotic surgery.

1585. France. European battlefield surgery surpasses Galen.

Galen's surgical works from the 2nd century AD were the standard textbooks during the Middle Ages in Western Europe. The use of gunpowder and shot was first introduced at the Battle of Crecy in 1346, it caused appalling wounds about which Galen's experience and writings naturally had nothing to contribute. The self-tutored and practical military surgeons of the time began to search for new ways to treat the wounded and in so doing began to weaken the existing uncritical belief in Galen.

Ambrose Paré[1] (1510–1590), a French barber-surgeon from Paris, published his *Oeuvres* (Works) in French rather than Latin in 1585. He had considerable experience of battlefield wounds and ligated bleeding arteries and veins as first practiced by Celsus[2] (c25 BC–c50 AD).

He also noticed that soldiers, who had been shot, frequently developed gangrene. This was blamed on gunpowder that was declared to be poisonous. In an effort to destroy the 'poison', it became the practice to pour boiling oil into the wounds or use red-hot cautery. Following one battle, there were so many wounded that Paré ran out of boiling oil. The following day, he found those treated with boiling oil in agony, while those who had escaped this treatment were much more comfortable[3]. He published this information and boiling oil was abandoned. The power of the printing press was now being recognised.[4]

Gangrene that developed in the wounds must have been caused by Clostridia perfringens,[5] a deadly gas forming organism that later became all too familiar in the trench warfare of the First World War.

A century after Paré's experience, Richard Wiseman (c1621–1680), an English surgeon, advised the immediate removal of the bullet with its accompanying 'rags' that had also been driven into the wound.[6] This method of treatment remained controversial through the Middle Ages.

References:

1. *A History of Surgery.* By Harold Ellis. Greenwich Medical Media Ltd, 2001.
2. Chapter 2. c30 AD. Celsus.
3. *A History of Surgery.* By Harold Ellis. Greenwich Medical Media Ltd, 2001.
4. Chapter 2. 1440. Books printed in Europe.
5. Wikipedia, Gas gangrene.
6. *Several Chirurgical Treatises by Richard Wiseman (1686).* Printed by R. Norton and F. Macock at the Ship in St Paul's Churchyard. Reproduction by Henry E. Huntingdon, Library and Art Gallery.

1609. Italy. The compound microscope developed by Galileo Galilei.

This is an example of technological advancement by Galileo Galilei (1564–1642). He was an Italian polymath who invented a telescope, thermometer and microscope. The originality of the microscope was that it had both convex and concave lenses.[1] Galileo's microscope was probably the first with two lenses and earlier than that of Zacharias Janssen (c1585–c1632) who between 1590 and 1618 also claimed to have invented a microscope. It is not clear who had the primacy.[2]

The microscope also became a tool of inestimable value in furthering the understanding of nature and the advancement of medicine. It was a bridge between anatomy and physiology. Its use proved the existence of capillaries, fed by the arteries and drained by the veins. These observations were the final confirmation of Dr William Harvey's proof of the circulation of the blood.[3]

References:

1. *The Cambridge Illustrated History of the Worlds Science.* By Colin A. Ronan. Book Club associates, Cambridge University Press, 1983, p 375.
2. Wikipedia. Zacharias Janssen.
3. Dr William Harvey See entry below.

1628. England. William Harvey and the circulation of the blood.

Dr William Harvey[1] (1588–1658) was a Fellow of the College of Physicians of London, also Physician to St Bartholomew's Hospital in London and sometime physician to both King James the First and King Charles the First of the United Kingdom. In 1628, he published his account of the circulation of the blood in *De Motu*

Cordis and *De Circulatione Sanguinis.*

Harvey was an expert anatomist and had dissected over forty species of animals which included birds and reptiles. He studied in detail the circulation of the blood and found that the heart was best studied when functioning. He measured the quantity of blood expelled with each heartbeat in a small animal and also the number of heartbeats in half an hour. The total capacity of the heart studied (converted into metric numbers) was 43 ml and of this 4.7 ml was ejected with each heartbeat. He estimated there were approximately one-thousand beats every half hour. The total volume of blood, pumped out of the heart every half hour was 4.7 litres and in 24 hours, the volume pumped was 225 litres.[2] This quantity of blood, pumped from a small heart, is incompatible with the ancient idea of the blood flowing up and down the arteries and veins with the blood being consumed in each organ. The only explanation was that blood circulated as Harvey proposed.

In other experiments to confirm this, he showed that tying the vena cava where it enters the right atrium of the heart resulted in a build-up of blood in the veins, while the ventricles and arteries emptied. He also demonstrated that blood pumped from the left ventricle into the arteries then passed through all the tissues of the body, to reach the veins and then return to the heart. He demonstrated that tying the great arteries near the heart caused it to swell as blood returned to the heart through the veins. This one-way flow of blood in the arteries and veins was also confirmed, in his well-known demonstration, that blood in the veins always flows towards the heart and backflow was prevented in the limbs by the venous valves.[3] With this proof that blood circulated, he postulated the presence of capillaries in the tissues. It was not long afterwards that these were identified by Marcello Malpighi (1628–1694) while studying the lung of a frog under a microscope.

Harvey had studied at the University of Padua in Italy in 1598 and attended the lectures of Hieronymus Fabricius[4] (1537–1619), the Professor of Anatomy who was also a surgeon. Fabricius was perfecting his knowledge of the anatomy of the valves in the veins that he had rediscovered in 1584. He published a treatise *De Venarum Osteolis* in 1603 that showed the existence of the venous valves. He demonstrated this to his students and there is no doubt that Harvey knew this. However, Fabricius misinterpreted the function of the valves believing that they prevented over distension of the veins when blood passed from the larger veins to the smaller. This is of course the reverse of what actually happens, his second error was to think that the absence of valves in the arteries confirmed the idea of the ancients that blood flowed down and then returned back up them.

In spite of his eminent position in London, Harvey's publication of *De Motu Cordis* was criticised and he was ostracised by contemporary physicians. Many continued to believe for some decades that Galen's description of the blood going up and down the arteries was correct. Harvey's medical practice was damaged by these criticisms and is an illustration that wrong but entrenched beliefs are difficult and take time to change.

References:

1. *William Harvey. 1578–1657.* By D'Arcy Power to Dr Philip Pye-Smith, F.R.S. in recognition of his profound knowledge of the Principles Advocated by Harvey. May 20th 1897. Reprinted in Britain by Amazon. ISBN 9781546334590.
2. The *Anatomical Exercises. De Motu Cordis and De Circulatione Sanguinis.* By William Harvey, 1628. Edited by Geoffrey Keynes. Republished by Dover Publications Inc. New York. 1995.
3. *The Heart and Vascular System in Ancient Greek Medicine. From Alcmaeon to Galen,* by C.R.S. Harris. Oxford University Press, 1983, special edition 2001, ISBN 0-19-858135-1, (The Chapter on Galen gives a masterly summary of the heart and blood in antiquity).
4. *Andreas Vesalius, the Reformer of Anatomy.* James Moores Ball. Saint Louis USA. Medical Science Press. 1910. Republished 2017 Trieste Publishing Pty Ltd, p 16 & 51.

c1650s. France. Partial excision of the tongue.

This was the second original operation of this medieval period and the earliest successful attempt to perform a partial glossectomy. This was by Dr Pimpernelle, who died in 1658. Little is known about him and the authority for this operation was given by Sir Frederick Treaves[1] quoting from 'Holmes System of Surgery' of 1883.

In 1758, an English surgeon, Mr Gutherie, is thought to be the first to excise a cancer of the tongue. This was followed in 1803 by Dr Inglis who removed a part of the tongue by strangulation with a ligature and Dr Chassaignac in 1854 who used an éccraseur, (a wire or fine chain cutter).[2] These were all partial glossectomies.

The first total glossectomy was by Dr Mirault in 1833. This proved successful because he ligated the lingual arteries and so prevented torrential and sometimes fatal haemorrhage during the operation. The operation itself is complex and as in all operations, detailed knowledge of anatomy is essential.

Glossectomy for cancer is often accompanied by a block dissection of the associated lymph nodes.[3]

References:

1. *A Manual of Operative Surgery*. By Sir Frederick Treves and Jonathon Hutchinson Volume 2. Lea and Febiger, 1910. Reprinted by Forgotten Books 2017.
2. *Ibid. Use of an éccraseur, (a wire or fine chain cutter).*
3. *Bailey and Love's Short Practice of Surgery.* By A.J. Harding Rains and H. David Richie. 17th Edition London H.K. Lewis and Co Ltd. 1987.

1665. England. First publication and wide distribution of learned medical journals.

The Royal Society of London was founded in 1660 and was the first Learned Society to regularly publish a journal. The first edition of the *Philosophical Transactions* was produced in 1665 when it carried articles by celebrated names in science and medicine.

Between 1673 and 1680, *Acta Medica et Philosophica Hafniensia* was published in Denmark by Dr Thomas Batholin (1616–1680). This journal also included articles on zoology and botany. In the USA, the *Medical Repository* was published in 1798[1] and the *Edinburgh Medical Journal* was published in 1802. It was followed by the *Lancet* in England in 1803. These and many other journals enabled standard practice and new procedures to be rapidly discussed and disseminated.[2]

References:

1. Wikipedia. The Medical Repository, USA.
2. *A History of Surgery.* By Harold Ellis. Greenwich Medical Media Ltd. 2001, ISBN 1 84110 023 4.

1673. Netherlands. Identification of bacteria.

Anthoni van Leeuwenhoek (1632–1723) was a Dutchman who manufactured his own microscope and was the first microbiologist. He drew pictures of his discoveries. One was of bacteria collected from his mouth. After initial scepticism, his work was fully accepted by the Royal Society of London who made him a fellow. He corresponded regularly with the Royal Society until his death.

Reference:

1. Wikipedia. Anthoni van Leewenhoek.

1740. France. The first skin transplant.

In 1740, Dr Garengeot, a French physician, reconstructed a soldier's nose using skin from another part of the body.[1] This differs from the original plastic surgical operations described by Sushruta in c200 BC. This is because Sushruta's skin pedicles remained attached to their origins, so maintaining an existing blood supply.[2] Dr Garengeot, therefore, described the first transplant, where skin was completely removed from the donor site to be transplanted elsewhere. This was the third original operation of this period.

Professor Karl Thiersch (1822–1895), Professor of Surgery in Leipzig, described in 1874 his method of using a thin superficial film of epidermis taken from the patient using a specialised blade. This thin layer of skin was used to cover large areas of burns on the same patient, reducing fluid loss and facilitating rapid healing. Thiersch's dermatome for harvesting skin is still used and bears his name.[3]

Reference:

1. *Organ Transplantation.* By Peter Petechuck. Greenwood Press, Westport USA. 2006, ISBN 0-313-33542-7.
2. Chapter 2. c200 BC. Sushruta.
3. *A History of Surgery*. By Harold Ellis. Greenwich Medical Media Ltd. 2001.

1768. England. The development of Teaching Hospitals in London.

Independent charitable hospitals began to teach students surgery in the 18th century. After the Edict of Tours of 1163, the teaching of surgery at universities ceased and by the 14th century surgical training was only by apprenticeship.

The development of how formal teaching of surgery in hospitals started can be illustrated by Mr John Hunter (1728–1793) following his appointment as a surgeon to the 200 bedded St George's Hospital in London in 1768.[1] The rules for the hospital's four surgeons demanded that, 'They attend to see all their patients twice a week. There were to be no operations, except for accidents, except on Mondays, Wednesdays and Fridays. On each of these days, dressings or operations were permitted between 11 am and 1 pm'. It was then the practice for surgeons to operate on more wealthy patients in their homes. A list of the operations that Hunter performed is given in Chapter 12, and consisted of his copying the original operations of the Ancient Egyptians and Greeks, to these he added his own original operation of parotidectomy.[2 & 3]

The surgical schedule at St George's with only six hours a week for operating, confirms that the hospital's surgical load was light. It must have been sufficient for operations such as drainage of abscesses and amputations. Pupils had to be on the wards to, 'Learn a sufficient knowledge of their profession (that) cannot be acquired without a constant and daily attendance'. This brought St Georges into line with St Thomas's and Guys' Hospital that had 700 beds, St Bartholomew's 400 and the London Hospital 140. The curriculum included midwifery, surgery, pharmacology with the practice of medicine, chemistry and anatomy. From now on surgery was also taught on a collegiate basis in the hospitals of London, all of them were independent charitable foundations without university connections.

From Hunter's time, the Teaching Hospitals accepted pupils to study surgery without a medical degree, giving them the opportunity to learn the science and practice of surgery at the highest level. At the same time, surgeons were also increasing their influence by joining together as the Barber-Surgeons of London and then through several stages were elevated to become the Royal College of Surgeons of England by Royal Charter in 1843.

By these means, surgeons through their own efforts had now established the organisational infrastructure to train surgeons and examine and licence them to practice. The ultimate prize for a young surgeon became and still is, to be awarded a Fellowship by the Royal College of Surgeons.

Some universities did begin to teach the science of surgery at undergraduate level. Sir Thomas Clifford Allbutt (1836–1925), when Regius Professor of Physic at Cambridge, wrote that when he was awarded his degree of Bachelor of Medicine from Cambridge University in 1861, he was only given a certificate that he had attended surgical lectures. Surgery was still not then recognised as fit to be a degree course.[4] It is astonishing to think that the Edict of Tours of 1163 had prevented physicians and surgeons from joining together to teach both subjects at University during the previous seven centuries.

Surgeons during this time had initially organised themselves through Guilds, later to provide training through the use of apprenticeships followed by the development of Teaching Hospitals, while the Royal College of Surgeons was responsible for examining candidates before permitting them to practise independently.

So, seven hundred years after the *Edict of Tours* and half a century after Allbutt's revelation, both medicine and surgery were reunited as degree courses at a number of universities. The Teaching Hospitals were incorporated into both the National Health Service and Universities in the UK in 1947. The Royal College of Surgeons kept its independence and continues to examine surgeons, ensuring that the highest standard of practice is maintained.

References:

1. *John Hunter Man of Science and Surgeon. Masters of Medicine.* By Stephen Paget, Sir James Paget & Ernest Hart. Leopold Classic Library. First printed in 1847. P 92.
2. Parotidectomy. John Hunter's original operation. See entry immediately below.
3. Chapter 2. c170 AD, Antyllus.
4. *The Historical Relations of Medicine and Surgery to the End of the Sixteenth Century.* Thomas Clifford Allbutt. Address delivered at the St Louis Congress in 1904. Hard Press Publishing USA.

1785. England. The first parotidectomy.

Mr John Hunter (1728–1793) was the most famous British surgeon of the 18th century, who carried out an original operation at a time when they were rare. He excised a bulky parotid tumour.[1] It weighed 1.2 kg and measured 23 x 17.5 centimetres and was excised without complications on the 24th of October 1785. This was a superficial parotidectomy and the facial nerve[2] was not damaged. This was the fourth original operation in this period.

In 1805, Dr George McClellan (1849–1913), Professor of Surgery at Thomas Jefferson Medical College, USA, performed a series of thirty parotidectomies of which 11 were for carcinoma with the facial nerve being deliberately sacrificed. One patient died due to the inadvertent ligature of the common carotid artery. McClellan published a textbook, the '*Principles and Practice of Surgery*' in 1848.[3]

In 1825, Dr Johann Ferdinand Heyfelder, a German surgeon at Erlangen, was the first to preserve the facial nerve during a parotidectomy for cancer.

By the 1950s, superficial parotidectomy with facial nerve identification and preservation was the standard operation. By the beginning of the 21st century, a more conservative approach, known as an extra capsular dissection, has had better postoperative results when carried out in high-volume centres. There was also a reduction of post-operative facial nerve palsy and Frey's syndrome. The latter condition is due to disruption of the auricular-temporal nerve, that causes sweating and flushing near the ear. These modern advances have reduced the length of time that patients stay in hospital.[4]

References:

1. Royal College of Surgeons of England. On line collections. *Salivary adenoma. Excised by John Hunter in 1785.*
2. A Brief History of Salivary Gland Surgery. Onivaldo Cervantes *et al.,* Rev. Col. Bras. Vol 44 no. 4 Rio de Janeiro July/August 2017. On line version ISSN 1809–4546.
3. Wikipedia. George McClellan (physician).
4. *Parotid Gland Surgery for Benign Tumours: Have we Come Full Circle.* By Dennis Yu Kim Chua, Christopher Hood and Keng Goh. Dept. of Otolaryngology Singapore General Hospital. Journals.sagepub.com 201010581402300109. Review.

1799. England. The Hunterian Museum at the Royal College of Surgeons of England.

The Hunterian Museum[1] was named after John Hunter (1728–1793), who was a Scottish surgeon who practised in London. He began his career dissecting and lecturing at Dr William Hunter's school of anatomy[2] and later established his own school. Dr Hunter was John's older brother. Whenever possible John Hunter dissected and studied daily and carried out physiological experiments. Many of his specimens have been preserved and can be seen in the Hunterian Museum at the Royal College of Surgeons of England. His collections include artefacts and dissections of man and animals from all over the world. His interests included comparative anatomy and among his dissections were exotic specimens brought back by Sir Joseph Banks (1743–1820), who had travelled round the world with Captain James Cook (1728–1779) in HMS Endeavour between 1768 and 1771.[3]

Hunter's specimens demonstrate the importance of structure to function as well as the similarity of all animals. In one series of exhibits, he compared the neurology of the earthworm with other animals including man. Hunter was on the right path but did not make an evolutionary connection. That was left to Mr Charles Darwin(1809-1882) and Mr Alfred Wallace Russell (1823-1913) whose papers on evolution were both presented at a meeting of the Linnean Society of London in 1858.[4] Darwin's great work *On the Origin of Species* was published a year later. Genetic studies have now proved the close relationship that exists between all living creatures. Unfortunately, not all the artefacts of Hunter's detailed and brilliant anatomical and surgical experiments have survived the depredations of time and war, but those that survive are important exhibits.

References:

1. The Royal College of Surgeons of England, Lincolns Inn Fields, London.
2. *The Knife Man: Blood, Body-snatching and the birth of modern Surgery.* By Wendy Moore: Bantam Books 2005.
3. *Voyages of Discovery. Three Centuries of Natural History Exploration.* By Dr Tony Rice. 1999. The Natural History Museum, London. ISBN 1-902686-02-0.

4. The Linnean Society of London. https://www.linnean.org

1809. USA. First planned laparotomy, the excision of an ovarian cyst.

This was the 5th and last original operation of this period. In 1809, Dr Ephraim McDowell (1771–1830), an Edinburgh trained doctor who practiced in Danville, Kentucky in the USA, was called to see a Mrs Crawford who thought she was in labour at the age of 44. McDowell travelled 60 miles to her home on horseback. His physical examination revealed a large abdominal swelling situated more to the left side of the abdomen. Vaginal examination revealed a normal cervix and an empty uterus. He diagnosed a huge ovarian cyst and said that if the patient could come to his house, he would perform an 'experiment'. Mrs Crawford presented herself a week later.

The operation was successful in removing a huge left ovarian cyst through a left paramedian abdominal incision. She returned home 25 days later. The operation was without any strong analgesia and of course, there was no anaesthetic at that date. This was an original operation on a brave woman.

McDowell waited to publish his results until 1817, by which time he had successfully carried out two more such operations, in all he did 13. His primacy, as the first surgeon ever to undertake an elective laparotomy was eventually accepted by his colleagues, who then acknowledged him as the 'father of abdominal surgery'. Mrs Crawford and her husband moved to Indiana, where she was elected as a state representative in the legislature and died aged 78.[1]

This first laparotomy was an original operation and also a seminal milestone in the progress of surgery. Before McDowell carried out this successful laparotomy, the abdomen had not been opened electively. Trauma by sword or other weapon that had exposed the abdominal cavity and its contents has occurred from the beginning of human conflict. Surgeons of their time did their best, but death was the usual outcome of such wounds due to sepsis. Hippocrates[2] (460–370 BC) when operating on inguinal hernias was aware of this and took care not to enter the abdomen for fear of causing suppuration and death.

From 1846, following the availability of anaesthesia, oophorectomy was popularised by Mr Spencer Wells[3] (1818–1898) in Britain. By 1871, he had carried out over 800 hundred such operations with a mortality of 25%. By 1876, the mortality following the introduction of Lister's antiseptic technique of surgery had fallen to 11%.

Why Mrs Crawford's wound did not become infected was probably due to McDowell's rural practice in a sparsely populated area where pathogenic organisms were rare. Compare this to Spencer Wells' frightening initial mortality of 25%, when the operations took place, in an as yet unrecognised pathogen infested hospital, in a city when infection was common and usually fatal. The subsequent fall in mortality to 11% by 1871 was a great improvement following the introduction of the antiseptic surgical technique devised by Professor Joseph Lister[4] in 1865. A few years later, other surgeons started using the strictly aseptic method while operating and reduced the mortality to 6%. In modern times, a patient dying from this operation would be a tragic rarity.

References:

1. *A History of Surgery*. By Harold Ellis. Greenwich Medical Media Ltd. 2001, ISBN 1 84110 023 4.
2. Chapter 2. c425 BC, Hippocrates.
3. *Seventy Years of Abdominal Surgery.* By Sir Zachary Cope, Science Medicine and History. Essays on the evolution of scientific thought and medical practice. Volume Two. Oxford University Press 1953.
4. Chapter 2. 1865, Joseph Lister.

1840s. Poland. The rise of therapeutic nihilism and the hope of new philosophy of medicine.

The rise of therapeutic nihilism, especially in medicine, began in the 1840s. Physicians were recognising that the decoctions and infusions listed in the pharmacopoeias and used for medical treatment were often useless or actually harmful. Perhaps this was an echo of the situation in Ancient Egypt nearly four thousand years earlier.

A physician who understood this was Dr Joseph Dietl (1804–1878) of Krakow, Poland. He taught his students that they could not develop panaceas or banish death but must discover why people became ill, through the scientific study of disease.

These sentiments could apply equally well to surgery, for it was a fact that an untold number of patients died, who suffered from conditions that are now treatable. Among these are strangulated hernias, rupture of ectopic pregnancies, infants with pyloric stenosis, obstruction to the gut from tumours and the list could go on. All of these conditions eventually became treatable following the introduction of anaesthetics in 1846.

Reference:

1. *The Cambridge Illustrated History of Medicine.* Edited by Roy Porter. Cambridge University Press 1996. 138 & 142.

Chapter 11

Analysis of Surgery in the Fourth Period

1. Introduction.
2. The devastating effect on surgery caused by the Edict of Tours of 1163.
3. The progress of medieval and early modern surgeons and surgery.
4. The development of Teaching Hospitals in Great Britain.
5. From Apprenticeship to Fellowship of the Royal College of Surgeons of England.
6. Philosophers in the Middle Ages separate of science from religion, leading to advances in technology and resurgence of surgery
7. Summary.

1. Introduction

This fourth period was remarkable for producing only five original operations and the first of these did not take place for nearly 1300 years after the last original operation. The principle reason being the comprehensive number of original operations undertaken by the Ancient Egyptians, Greeks and Indians. There were contributory reasons for the absence of original operations in Byzantium and the Caliphates of Baghdad and Cordova that have already been presented. This period looks at the continuing lack of original operations that only ended in 1575. For it was also a period of great endeavour both intellectual and practical that laid the basis for the huge advances of the fifth and last period of original operations

2. The devastating effect of the Edict of Tours of 1163.

The 'Edict of Tours' caused a dramatic change for the worse in the practice of surgery when Pope Alexander III[1] in 1163 pronounced, 'Ecclesia Abhorret a Sanguine'. Loosely translated, it means that the church was opposed to the shedding of blood by the clergy. This was interpreted by them to apply not only to fighting in battle, but also to the practice of surgery. This may, or may not, have been an unintended consequence of the Edict, but the result was disastrous.

It has been disputed that the Pope made any such pronouncement. However, Canon 8 of the Edict of Tours specifically prohibited clerics from involving themselves in studies of a physical nature. The pope had declared that anyone undertaking such studies, 'Must be in league with the Devil'. Physicians were all university educated and were also in those days part of the clergy, even if not ordained as priests. They were now forbidden to carry out any physical labour. They considered that operating fell into that category and decided that they could proceed to abandon surgery, which was precisely what they did.[2]

The effect was summed up by Professor Clifford T. Allbutt, Regius Professor of Physic at Cambridge University who during a lecture he gave in 1904 in the USA bluntly said, "Medicine had lopped off its right arm by the expulsion of surgery from the liberal arts, when this pernicious bisection of medicine was made." He went on to say, 'Surgery, hated and avoided by Medical Faculties, scorned in clerical and feudal circles, (now) began in the hands of lowly and uneducated men to grow from the root.'[3]

In this way, the barbers, shavers and haircutters, who before the edict had been delegated by the clergy to perform minor surgical procedures such as venesection and lancing of abscesses were now by default in charge of the whole practice of surgery and left to fend for themselves.[4] The status of surgeons had now reached its lowest point.

The effect of completely separating surgery from medical practice was both profound and illogical. Illogical because surgery had always been the active and practical arm of medicine and in the times of the Ancient Egyptians was more advanced than medicine, for medicine was then dominated by magic. Now, forbidden entry to the universities on account of both their class and lack of education, the barbers and surgeons during the subsequent centuries gradually began to organise themselves.

This started in 1252 when a Guild of Barber-Surgeons was founded in Montpellier and of course they were not associated with the University in that city. Guilds followed in Paris in 1260 and London in about 1300. The Guilds were very powerful in the Middle Ages and as they were incorporated by Royal Charter, they could admit new members and maintain standards and discipline in their crafts. Those dismissed from their guild were no longer permitted to practise. The very limited number of operations that it was possible to practice at that time were all existing original operations, from the first and second periods of surgery.

In Medieval Europe, people who followed the same craft or trade tended to live near each other or even in the same street. This enabled competition to be regulated, standards to be maintained and the spiritual and material welfare of their members to be looked after. In 1308, nearly 150 years after the Edict of Tours, the Barber's Company of London[5] was first mentioned, when Richard le Barbour was elected as an Alderman in 1308 to preside over it. The Barber's Company included surgeons from 1312. It was unclear whether the surgeons were also barbers who had decided to specialise, as their duties at that time overlapped. A great advance was when apprenticeships were started. The trainee surgeons then worked for between five and seven years under a member of the Barber's Company who controlled and supervised them.

In 1416, a Guild of Surgeons[6] was approved. This led to disputes between the Barber's Company and the Guild, resulting in the Barbers Company being given the power to regulate the surgeons, thereby indicating just how far the status of surgeons had fallen. A new Act of Parliament in 1547, decreed that individual members could be either barbers or surgeons, but not both when they became the Company of Barber-Surgeons.[7] This Charter was also necessary because unqualified persons, 'not sufficiently skilled', have created, 'almost infinite evils'. The damage done to the reputation of surgery by unqualified men was lamented by the surgeon Thomas Gale.[8]

Throughout this time, the philosophic and medical treatises of Hippocrates and Galen continued to be studied in the universities, while surgery continued to be ignored. The Barber Surgeons fended for themselves and the question arises whether they had access to the detailed surgical texts of the Ancient Greeks and Romans, or were they having to struggle to establish a primitive level of surgery by themselves?

For surgery, unlike philosophy, was and is a practical craft, good descriptions of operations that had been carried out and described in antiquity could be followed and copied to the advantage of both surgeons and patients. For if it was found that the surgical treatises of Hippocrates and Galen were available and literally within their grasp, this would be of the utmost importance in guiding them to begin the long haul to reach the standards of Ancient Greek surgery.

To help in this search, books written by a series of medieval surgeons who practiced in England and France and wrote of their experience give us an insight of what happened.

3. Medieval and early modern surgeons.

The first notable surgeon of this time was John of Arderne[9] (1307–1392), an Englishman who was considered the first to bring Hippocrates' original operation for treating anal fistulae to England. He wrote on both medicine and surgery and had been a student at Montpellier University and when there had access to Hippocrates' treatises including his description of the operation for curing fistulae-in-ano. Dr Donald Campbell informs us that Arderne himself transcribed from the Arabised texts.[10] It was later wrongly claimed in England that Arderne was the originator of the operation to cure fistulas-in-ano, but as we know that accolade belongs to Hippocrates.[11]

Gunpowder and shot were introduced and first used in Europe in 1346 at the Battle of Crecy. Canons were soon to be followed by handguns. Naturally, Galen's surgical treatises had nothing to contribute concerning the management of the wounds they caused. This for the first time, engendered doubts concerning Galen's infallibility.

In 1514, Giovanni da Vigo[12] (1450–1525) an Italian Surgeon, wrote on how to treat gunshot wounds. He believed that gunpowder was the cause of gangrene that frequently developed in these wounds. To counteract this 'poison', he recommended treating the wounds with red hot cautery or by pouring boiling oil into them. There was no evidence that this helped, but despite this, the book he wrote on the subject was popular and ran to 54 editions. This barbaric treatment resulted in many wounded soldiers suffering serious additional injury during this low point in surgical practice.

When in 1537, Ambroise Paré[13] (1510–1590), a Frenchman and skilled barber-surgeon, attended the wounded at the Battle of Turin, he treated gun-shot wounds by pouring boiling oil into them as had been advised by Vigo. He did not have enough boiling oil for the last few wounded and worried about his inability to treat these patients. Early next morning when he went to review them, he found those treated with boiling oil to be feverish and in agony, while those he had only been able to treat with simple medicaments were comfortable and their wounds looked more settled following the treatment they had received.

Box 11.1.

The 1st Original operation of this fourth period was by Ambroise Paré, when in 1575 he, performed a trans-urethral prostatectomy.[13]

These text boxes have been introduced to draw attention to each of the five original operations in this fourth period of surgery. Also, other boxes show the operations performed by individual and named medieval surgeons. It must be noted that apart from the five original operations of this Period, of which this was the first, all the other operations practised originated in Antiquity.

He wrote of his experiences so that soldiers could be spared from boiling oil. Paré had acted on the empirical evidence before him, his fame grew and he was later appointed Surgeon to the King of France.

Other discoveries that loosened the grip of the Ancients were taking place. In 1543, learning by experiment and observation was given a boost by two eminent scientists in very different spheres of learning. Nicolaus Copernicus (1473–1543)[14] published in the year of his death, *On the Revolution of the Celestial Spheres*. In which he proved the 'Heliocentric theory' that the sun was the centre of the universe. This caused consternation to the huge majority of people who still believed the Greek theory that the Earth was the centre of the Universe as laid down by Pythagoras.

In the same year, Andreus Vesalius (1514–1564)[15] professor of Anatomy at the University of Padua in Italy, published, *On the Fabric of the Human Body*, in Latin. This was the first textbook of whole-body anatomy, made from his direct observations while dissecting human cadavers. The sporadic dissections of humans in Italy over the previous two centuries had added some new knowledge, but it was still Galen's dissections of animals, principally macaques, from over 1300 years earlier that were finally superseded by Vesalius.

Then in 1563, Thomas Gale[16] (1507–1587) published a book, *Certaine Vvorks of Chirurgerie.* In its first Chapter, he discusses with another surgeon and a friend the state of surgery in England at that time. He was worried about the poor reputation of surgeons, caused by men who had set themselves up to practise surgery without any training. This was at a time when a lengthy apprenticeship was the proper entry to the profession.

Gale then asks his friends whether they have read the works of Hippocrates, Galen, Paul of Aegina and Rhazes, all of whom he had studied. By referring to these authors, Gale demonstrates that, despite the Edict of Tours, surgeons were now in possession of and strongly influenced by the original operations described and practiced by the Ancient Greeks already in Latin and about this time beginning translated into English by John of Arderne.[10] Gale goes on to lament that, "Chirurgerie (surgery) is so joined to medicine and physic (medicine) that it cannot be well separated from them, though they are now two different arts. Truth it is (that) in the beginning (of the practice of medicine and surgery), physic and chirurgerie were both one, and one man exercised both, as did the princes of physic Hippocrates and Galen. Thus, I perceive that chirurgerie is not so base as it is taken for, and that it is of great antiquity, being the most authentic part of physic and was exercised by emperors, kings, philosophers and physicians."

Box 11.2.
The operations of Thomas Gale[8]. 1507–1587. All were practised in Antiquity except for Gunshot wounds.

1. Excision of skin tumours.
2. Setting fractures.
3. Reducing dislocations.
4. Venesections.
5. Trephination of the skull.

He then goes on to give Galen's definition of surgery. 'Chirurgirie is a part of therapeutics, healing men by incision and articulation. But also (healing) by physic, which cures by diet, medicines or by using their head (brain).'

Gale had investigated the controversy of whether gunpowder was poisonous or not. He had never used boiling oil as a 'treatment' for gunshot wounds, but knew that gunpowder was manufactured from sulphur, saltpetre and coal. Referring to Galen's pharmacopoeia he found that these substances were listed and all were considered harmless when used to treat wounds and ulcers. Gale published these findings to let it be known that gunpowder was not a poison.

If we now examine Gale's surgical practice, in Box 11.2, it shows that apart from wounds caused by gunshot, that were not usually operated upon, all the other operations he carried out were original operations from Peru, Ancient Egypt and Greece.

Gale taught that if a soldier had been shot in the abdomen, it was better to leave the shot inside rather than increase the damage trying to find it. He had been influenced not to operate by his observation that any abdominal organ penetrated by shot resulted in the soldier's death. How to treat gunshot wounds remained controversial until the First World War when active debridement and leaving wounds open to drain freely became the norm. It is of note that the range of operations practiced by Gale was significantly less than those of the Ancients.

The next medieval surgeon of interest was Richard Wiseman[17] (1622–1676), whose book, *Several Chirugrical Treatises*, was published in the year of his death. He fought in the English Civil Wars and became Surgeon and Sergeant-Surgeon to King Charles II. His treatises are of particular interest as they contain many case histories of patients in war and peace. He began to serve as an apprentice in 1637 and was afterwards admitted to the Guild of Barber-Surgeons of London when Henry Blackey was Master in the same year.[18] Wiseman had accepted Dr William Harvey's proof of the circulation of the blood before many of his colleagues.

In this respect, he was modern, but as with all doctors and surgeons, he was still bound within the Hippocratic framework for the practice of medicine and surgery in the absence of knowing the cause of disease. Wiseman continued to starve, purge and bleed his patients. He was well read and quotes extensively from the works of Hippocrates, Celsus and Galen and other more contemporary surgeons.

Wiseman's operations are listed in Box 11.3. His case histories confirm that patients did not consult a surgeon until very late in their disease, probably for fear of the pain that an operation would cause. He ligated bleeding arteries as described by Celsus and may have been the first to attempt to sew the ends of a severed artery together. This was without success in two cases, his failure being almost certainly due to the crudity and size of his sutures and needles.

> **Box 11.3.**
>
> The operations of Richard Wiseman[17] 1622–1676. All are original operations from Antiquity except for Gunshot wounds.
>
> 1. Varicose veins.
> 2. Ligated bleeding arteries.
> 3. Cautery of small aneurysms.
> 4. Mastectomy.
> 5. Hydroceles.
> 6. Hernias.
> 7. Suture of severed tendons.
> 8. Trephination of the skull.
> 9. Fistula-in-ano.
> 10. Amputations.
> 11. Probing for shot in gunshot wounds.

Cancers of the breast presented late, usually with fixation to the underlying tissues. In the few women he operated on with this disease, he used cautery which caused terrible pain. A similar technique was used on a cancer of the rectum which was not successful and is not included as an original operation. His treatment for fistulae-in-ano was exactly as described by Hippocrates and he followed Galen in attempting to suture severed tendons. Wiseman trephined the skull for both civilian head injuries and war wounds and does not mention sepsis as a problem. All his operations apart from the treatment of gunshot wounds were original operations from antiquity.

With gunshot wounds, he emphasised the removal not only of the ball but also any pieces of clothing driven in with it. The controversy of how to treat this problem continued. Wiseman showed concern for soldiers with abdominal gunshot wounds knowing that nearly all would die and wrote, 'It is not consistent with religion or humanity to leave such people without help and sometimes one cures one'. Wiseman was an example of diligence, hard work and practical knowledge that made him an exemplary surgeon of his time.

> **Box 11.4.**
>
> The 2nd original operation of this fourth period took place in 1650 and consisted of a partial excision of the tongue. This was undertaken by Dr Pimpernelle[19] in France, about whom little is known. It was a bold operation considering the torrential bleeding that occurs when the tongue is excised if the lingual artery has not been ligated previously.

All books written by surgeons, almost into early modern times, had to be censored before being approved as suitable to be printed. There were two Censors, the Bishop of London and the Censors of the College of Physicians of London. This requirement confirmed the inferior position of surgeons in the medical hierarchy during the Middle Ages. An example of censorship was when Richard Wiseman published his book in 1672 on surgery during the Civil Wars in England. He records advances and improvements in surgery since the times of Vigo and Gale, but even so the approval of the Censors of College of Physicians was still mandatory and it was granted for this publication. Wiseman was not only deeply read in Hippocrates' works but also Galen's. As Gale had also found, these works were now available to surgeons. It also confirms the continuity, influence and importance of the works of the Ancient Greeks to the end of the Middle Ages.

Even so, surgery was still an unsophisticated craft and had made little if any advance on Galen. Few serious wounds or diseases of the limbs were curable; amputation was frequent and carried a high mortality.

At about the same time, Hippocrates' operation for cutting and removing a bladder stone through a perineal incision was being practised in London in 1658. A century later, Mr William Cheselden[20] (1687–1752) at St Thomas's Hospital in London could perform this operation in under two minutes. Again, there was emphasis on how essential it was to reduce the length of time an operation lasted to reduce death from shock. Cheselden published a series of 213 patients he had operated on to remove bladder stones with only twenty deaths. This was a remarkable record and the low mortality for that time indicates his skill and that sepsis in the then relatively small metropolis of London was not yet as dangerous as it was to become a century later.

Box 11.5.

The 3rd original operation of this fourth period was in 1740 and is the first recorded example of an autograft. It was by Dr Garengeot[21] a Frenchman about whom little else is known. He took a piece of skin from one part of the body and successfully transplanted it at another site on the same patient.

We can now focus on the last and most famous of the surgeons of the late Middle Ages and Early Modern period who was Mr John Hunter[22] (1728–1793) the foremost surgeon of the 18th century. He was a Scot who when he left school joined his brother Dr William Hunter (1718–1783), who was a physician, surgeon and anatomist in London. John became William Hunter's assistant and worked in his Anatomy School. John Hunter was fascinated by anatomy and would spend hours every day dissecting and preparing specimens for teaching. Through unsparing diligence, his knowledge of human and animal anatomy was eventually unrivalled and his fame spread to Europe. He also carried out many physiological experiments.

While serving with the army on Belle Isle off the coast of France, he carried out detailed studies on inflammation, sepsis and the treatment of wounds caused by gunshots. He advised against exploring the wounds 'because it increased the trauma and often fails to remove the ball and any material carried in'. He had seen materials that had been driven into wounds by a ball being naturally discharged along the bullet's tract many days later.[23]

Hunter's experiments included a detailed study of the development of a collateral circulation following the thrombosis of an aneurysm. From this, he deduced that ligating a functioning artery supplying an aneurysm would not precipitate gangrene in the limb beyond. He reasoned that such a ligation would cause connected arterioles, the collateral circulation, to dilate and carry an increasing flow of blood to the tissues beyond the aneurysm. In this, he was proved correct. For when he ligated a popliteal artery above an aneurysm that was about to burst, the leg below did not go gangrenous due to lack of a blood supply, as the collateral circulation opened up and the leg was saved. This may possibly have been an independent discovery and was acclaimed as an original operation at the time by others but not by Hunter himself.[24]

An interesting aside that follows, concerns the ligation of the artery that leads to an aneurysm beyond it, by Aetius of Amida[25] (502–575). In about 550, Aetius ligated the brachial artery above an aneurysm that was expanding at the elbow. It may be that both Aetius and Hunter arrived independently at the idea of ligating the artery feeding an aneurysm to prevent its rupture. This might demonstrate that when the same disease process is understood by different surgeons at different times, they may alight on the same treatment. It is possible that this was the case, especially as the technology available to them both, although separated by many centuries, was not dissimilar.

Box 11.6.

The operations of John Hunter[29] (1728–1793).

All we practised in antiquity except for gunshot wounds and his original operation of a parotidectomy.

1 Venesection.
2 Aneurysm, ligation of artery.
3 Achilles tendon sutures.
4 Trephination of the skull.
5 Varicose veins.
6 Hydrocele.
7 Orchidectomy.
8 Bladder stones.
9 Amputations.
10 Setting of fractures.
11 Dislocations.
12 Ligation of blood vessels.
13 Fistula-in-ano.
14 Incision of abscesses.
15 Mastectomy.
16 Hydrocele.
17 Caesarean section.
18 Hernia.

It is also possible that Hunter may have read Aetius's description of this operation. For Aetius' works were translated into Arabic from the Greek by Rhazes[26] and this was later translated into Latin by Gerard of Cremona (1114-1187) and quoted by Thomas Gale[27] in his book published in English in 1563.

It is unlikely that we will find a definite answer to this question, for the actual original operation of ligating an artery proximal to an aneurysm had taken place four centuries before that of Aetius by Antyllus,[28] who first carried it out in about 170 AD.

The operation having been performed in Antiquity leads one to speculate that as Hunter did not claim it as original operation, he was aware of its past history.

Hunter's surgical practise lies within the Hippocratic framework of disease, as the causes of diseases were still a mystery. So, despite his advances, he was bound, as were his predecessors, to the Hippocratic practice of surgery, as it was still relevant and could not yet be consigned to history.

Hunter[29] carried out a wide range of operations as shown in the Box 11.6 and it is significant that his 'general operations' were the original operations of the Ancients. He still practiced venesection, although reluctantly. However, like Antyllus, Hunter did become one of those very rare surgeons to definitely carry out an original operation, in his case a parotidectomy as shown in Box 11.7. Hunter continued with experiments to discover the function of organs and tissues on a scale not seen since the time that Dr William Harvey proved that blood circulated, and prepared the way for the modern era.

The question of whether the medieval and early modern surgeons had access to the writings of the ancient founders of surgery is now clearly in the affirmative. The books written by Thomas Gale and Richard Wiseman have quotes from Hippocrates, Galen, Celsus and others. The operations that Hunter carried out were also the original operations of the ancients. Adding these to his parotidectomy and the beginning of the rise of science, he paved the way for modern surgery just over half a century later.

Boxes 11.2, 11.3 and 11.6 list the operations performed by Gale, Wiseman and Hunter and show the steady increase in the number of the Ancients operations being undertaken by them between 1500 and 1800. There can be no doubt that the late medieval and early modern surgeons benefited from the descriptions of operations first performed in antiquity. So now, 600 years after the Edict of Tours of 1163, John Hunter's practice of surgery not only equalled those of the ancient surgeons, but had finally surpassed them with his original operation.

Box 11.7.

The 4th original operation of this fourth period of surgery was by John Hunter[30] in 1785 when he carried out a parotidectomy. He excised a huge benign parotid adenoma weighing four kilograms from John Burley without complications. Hunter recorded that Burley did not cry-out during the whole of the operation that lasted 25 minutes. Portraits of Burley before and after his operation are to be found in William Clift's catalogue at the Royal College of Surgeons of England.

4. The development of the Teaching Hospitals in London.

London's oldest hospitals are St Bartholomew's, founded in 1123 and St Thomas's Hospital, named after St Thomas Becket and founded after his death in 1173. It was not until the 18th century that four new hospitals were built and opened in London within the space of 24 years. These were Guy's Hospital in 1721, St Georges Hospital in 1733, the London Hospital in 1740 and the Middlesex Hospital in 1745. This rapid expansion was driven by the population of London trebling during the previous century from about 200,000 to nearly 600,000. At the same time, the city had increased in importance and prosperity. It was against this background that these hospitals, all charitable institutions, were formalising the teaching of surgery.

John Hunter was appointed as one of the four surgeons at St George's Hospital in 1768 where he and his colleagues taught surgical trainees. He gave lectures and took ward rounds to see his patients. He encouraged his students to attend daily to, 'gain sufficient knowledge of their profession'. This brought St George's into line with the other London teaching hospitals that now had a common curriculum that included midwifery, surgery, pharmacology and the teaching of physics, chemistry and anatomy. Hunter also began a course of lectures on the 'Principles and Practice of Surgery in 1793'.[31]

5. From medieval Guilds to the Royal College of Surgeons.

Not surprisingly, there were claims between the nations of Europe of which was pre-eminent in many fields of discovery including surgery. Between the onset of the two French Revolutions of 1789 and 1848, French revolutionary surgeons appointed to the hospitals in Paris, declared they were the leaders of medical education and 'Dominated its practice throughout the medical world'. They encouraged young surgeons to follow the military drum so as to learn the art of surgery first hand in battle.[32] Meanwhile in England in 1789, John Hunter had already been a surgeon and tutor at St Georges Hospital since 1768, 21 years earlier. It is also interesting that through the Middle Ages Messrs Arderne, Cope, Wiseman and Hunter had all followed the drum into battle to gain surgical experience, as had the French surgeon Amboise Paré before the Revolution. Perhaps the claims from Paris were only revolutionary propaganda!

In England, the standard of training advanced further when the apprenticeship was followed by an examination in surgery at the Hall of the Barber-Surgeons of London. To conduct this examination, a Court of Examiners of ten surgeons was formed and successful candidates became Freemen of the Company and were entitled to practice independently. By this time, those presenting themselves for examination had already served an apprenticeship and some had also attended more intensive training in a teaching hospital.

One such candidate in 1789 was Mr William Savory. He was examined at Surgeon's Hall following his apprenticeship and attendance at St Thomas' and Guys Hospitals. The courses at the Hospitals cost him £100, a considerable sum in those days. He passed the examination and later practiced as a surgeon in the town of Newbury.[33]

By Act of Parliament in 1745, the surgeons were separated from the barbers. The surgeons formed the Company of Surgeons. In 1800, the Company of Surgeons became the Royal College of Surgeons of London and finally in 1843 became the Royal College of Surgeons of England.[34]

As the system changed, apprenticeships were gradually abandoned after 1838, and by the late 19th century, the system had developed so that candidates could learn the basic sciences of anatomy, physiology and pathology at a Teaching Hospital, to be followed by three years as a surgical clerk in a hospital. Success in a new first examination then entitled them to practise surgery as a junior surgeon, limited to working in a hospital under supervision.

It was only then that young aspirants to the profession, having fulfilled the prescribed formal training followed by several years of practice under supervision, took a rigorous examination in all aspects of surgery at the Royal College of Surgeons. Successful candidates were awarded the prestigious Fellowship of the Royal College of Surgeons of England. A similar process took place at the Royal Colleges of Surgeons of Scotland and of Ireland.

At last, surgeons through their own efforts had elevated themselves from their lowly status following the Edict of Tours and had successfully established the organisational infrastructure to train, examine and licence surgeons to practise at the highest level.

There was still the matter of a lack of any university offering a degree in surgery to go alongside the existing degree of Batchelor of Medicine. Sir Thomas Clifford Allbutt[35] (1836–1925), then wrote that when he was awarded the

Cambridge degree of 'Bachelor of Medicine' in 1861, he had only been given a certificate to record that he had attended 'surgical lectures'.

The universities continued to ignore surgery as a fit subject to teach, until it was proposed by the University of London, founded in 1836, that first offered the degree of Batchelor of Surgery in 1863. Durham University also made a similar representation. At this point, the Royal College of Surgeons intervened and the universities were unable to proceed. This embargo did not last long and some universities began to award the degree of Batchelor of Surgery in the second half of the 19th century.

However, it remained that only the Royal College of Surgeons could grant a certificate, including a Fellowship to practice surgery independently to successful candidates after examination.[36] Students from 1863 onwards could now attend university to study for degrees in both medicine and surgery exactly 700 years after the Edict of Tours of 1163.

The numbers of Teaching Hospitals to train aspiring surgeons as well as physicians continued to increase throughout the United Kingdom of Great Britain and Ireland. These remained independent charitable institutions until they were incorporated into the National Health Service in the United Kingdom in 1948, it was then that they also became faculties of their local universities.

At last, the setback caused to surgery by the Edict of Tours in 1163 had finally been overcome. This long period of struggle explains why in Great Britain to this day surgeons are proud to call themselves Mister and not Doctor. This is in memory that their elevation to the status of trained qualified Surgeons had previously taken place without the benefit of a university degree. All surgeons now hold university degrees in both medicine and surgery or a qualification of equal standing.

Figure 11.8.

The 5th and last original operation of this fourth period of surgery was the first planned operation to be carried out within the abdominal cavity. It took place more than thirty years before the introduction of anaesthesia, when in 1809, Dr Ephraim McDowell[37] (1771–1830) an American country surgeon, who had trained at Edinburgh University, removed a large ovarian cyst, that he had correctly diagnosed preoperatively. His patient survived. She was an extraordinary woman who sang hymns throughout her operation.

6. Philosophers in the Middle Ages separate science from religion, leading to advances in technology and the resurgence of surgery.

In the 13th century, there were two trains of thought developing in Western Europe.

One was the start of new learning that was taking place, eventually to be known as science. This developed from the study of Aristotle's treatises in Latin translations, all of which were Arabised versions.

There was also a gradual realisation that the practice of medicine was not a vibrant exercise but had become an ossified dogma, in which the writings of Hippocrates and Galen had come to be believed as the final revelations on anatomy, medicine and surgery. From then onwards, dissatisfaction was growing with the idea that everything there was to be learnt concerning the practice of medicine and surgery had already been discovered in antiquity.

This change in outlook began when Robert Grosseteste[38] (1168–1253), a 'scholastic', who had lectured at Oxford and had been impressed by Aristotle's approach to the study of nature began to re-evaluate it. Grosseteste was the first to give a clear definition of science when he wrote, 'Science began with man's experience of phenomena. Its aims are to discover the reasons for this experience and to find the causes for it, then analyse them, reconstruct them as a hypothesis and finally verify or disprove them by further observation'. This definition is not out of place today.

Another advance was by Roger Bacon[39] (c1219–c1292), who had possibly been a pupil of Grosseteste and was following his own active interest in science. Bacon counter-intuitively described what he considered the four general causes of human ignorance that inhibited the development of science. These were, 'Frail and unsuitable authority, long custom, uninstructed popular opinion and concealment of ignorance in a display of apparent wisdom'. He believed that science led to knowledge and among his new interests was a study of optics. As Grosseteste had laid down the principles of science, Bacon had now described why it was so difficult for them to be accepted until Albertus Magnus[40] (1193–1280) re-evaluated them.

Albertus had read the 'Arabised' translations of Aristotle and was impressed, but did not join his contemporaries in considering Aristotle infallible. This was a significant intellectual break with traditional thinking. Albertus realised that Aristotle's philosophical writings were pagan and thought that a synthesis between Christian thought and that of Aristotle was needed. This followed the same line of thinking when in an earlier age, Aristotle's treatises had been aligned with Islam in the Arabic translations.

This new alignment was provided by St Thomas Aquinas[41] (1225–c1274), a Dominican friar who was sent to Paris to further his education under Albertus Magnus.

Thomas Aquinas later taught that in science, the Greeks had revealed the workings of God's world, but when it came to matters of salvation the Church and the Scriptures were the revealing authority. After his death, it was acknowledged that he had reconciled Christian orthodoxy and Greek science, leading to the Church gradually accepting this separation. St Thomas had risked much to come to this conclusion having spent fourteen years in prison for his beliefs.

It was left to John Dunn Scottus[42] (d 1308) to make the final separation of experiment and scientific reasoning from theology. He did this by understanding that higher spiritual knowledge was only attainable through inner awareness, because it did not involve the senses. This was in tune with Ancient Greek philosophy from the 7th century BC onwards. His train of thinking further facilitated the gradual separation of science from religion and ultimately reconciled independent human thought with the divine.

The subsequent growth in experimentation was a stepping-stone to the Scientific Revolution.

It was these intellectual advances that allowed the study of science and technological advances to flourish. This was underpinned by economic development that led to growth in the wealth of nations and ultimately to the Industrial Revolution.

Box 11.9.

How science and technology benefitted surgery.

1440.The introduction of the printing press.[43]

1506. The new science of pathological anatomy through regular post-mortems was beginning.[44]

1543. Vesalius' new anatomy textbook, *De Humani Corporis Fabrica*, derived directly from dissections of human cadavers was published. His discoveries significantly advanced anatomical learning and finally rendered Galen's anatomy redundant.[45]

1609. Galileo Gallileii developed the compound microscope.[46]

1628. William Harvey[47] published, *De Moto Cordis* and *Sanguinis Animalibus* proving the circulation of the blood. This was the greatest physiological advance since Galen's physiological experiments 1400 years earlier.

1665. Medical journals began regularly publication.[48]

1693. Bacteria were identified.[49]

1799. The first surgical museum was opened at the Royal College of Surgeons of London. The Hunterian Museum being a model of its kind.[50]

1846. The introduction of anaesthesia was the single greatest advance for surgery and made possible planned elective operations within the great cavities[51] of the body.

1846. The cause of sepsis was still unknown, but the reduction in sepsis following the washing of hands made it mandatory before examining a patient.[52]

For example, a great step forward was the identification of micro-organisms and the realisation that some of them are pathogens, leading to Lister's anti septic method of operating. This and many other factors led to the increasing safety of undergoing an operation.

7. Summary.

The reasons for only five original operations during this fourth period are now apparent. For the 38 original operations undertaken in antiquity had resulted in the superficial tissues of the body being comprehensively operated upon, for the ancients exhausted the possibility for further original operations until there were improvements in technology. Finer and better instruments were important in this respect. It was largely these that enabled innovative surgeons to undertake the five original operations of this period.

The Ancient Greeks through their philosophy had provided a framework, imperfect as it was, for the practice of both medicine and surgery. Their ideas survived the rise and fall of empires but could only develop and progress when the causes of diseases were discovered. We now know that the medieval and early modern surgeons had read the works of Hippocrates, Celsus and Galen, enabling them to copy the original operations of antiquity. These were the only operations practised between 180 and 1575, when the first original operation for over 1300 years took place.

Looking back, John Hunter in the 18th century can be considered the last of the great medieval surgeons. His surgical practice was still within the framework laid down by Hippocrates and even included his use of the malign treatment of venesection, even if only occasionally. John Hunter was more than this, he was also a scientist devoted to experimentation and the most learned anatomist of his day, many of his experiments can still be viewed in the Hunterian Museum at the Royal College of Surgeons of England in London. He was also elevated by being one of the only five surgeons to produce an original operation during this fourth period of surgery, when in 1785 he carried out a superficial parotidectomy.

The other surgeons who devised original operations in this period were Ambrose Paré in 1585, Dr Pimpernelle in 1650 and Dr Garengot in 1740. Then sixty-nine years later, within this same period, Dr Ephraim MacDowell in 1809 carried out, what had never been done before, a planned elective operation within the abdominal cavity before anaesthesia was introduced.

It was in this period that the damage done by the Edict of Tours was finally overcome, when at increasing pace surgeons developed a system for teaching surgery that grew in status and sophistication. This process had taken seven centuries before surgery was being practised at the highest level within the instrumentation and knowledge then available.

Without doubt, the Ancient Greek practice of surgery was dominant from the 5th century BC to the middle of the 19th century. The framework for practice devised by Hippocrates in an age before the causes of disease was known, regularised medical and surgical practice by establishing an intellectual framework within which to work. In these circumstances, his theories made sense despite all their inconsistencies. That extraordinary age has now been forgotten. It is worth reminding ourselves that nearly all the operations devised in antiquity are still practiced today, albeit much improved. The Greeks and other ancients left a unique legacy.

It also needs to be remembered how fragile the transfer of Greek manuscripts from one civilisation to the next had been. Many of the manuscripts of the ancient surgeons are lost, but a considerable literature survived and is available today. It was also fortuitous that Plato and Aristotle had monotheistic beliefs, that made their manuscripts of interest to Islamic scholars and made it possible for these scholars to align Plato's and Aristotle's works to the teachings of Islam, as they translated Greek manuscripts into Arabic. Without their philosophic beliefs, the Greek philosophy may not have been of interest to Arab scholars and have been forgotten. For it was Aristotle who wrote of the supreme, 'Unmoved Mover', in his belief of 'God as the eternal unchanging source of all change'.[53]

As it was the Arabised manuscripts translated into Latin were studied in Western Europe and venerated by the 'Scholastics' who incorporated them into the curricula of their universities and considered them unchangeable.

This stimulated the progression of brilliant scholars who over two centuries separated science from religion. Robert Grosseteste in the 13th century defined science, enabling Albertus Magnus in the same century to re-evaluate the philosophy of Plato and Aristotle in relation to Christianity, in the same way that it had been aligned with Islam. John Dunn Scottus, at the end of the same century separated science from theology, a fundamental step that enabled the Roman Catholic Church to countenance and tolerate the pursuit of science as a separate discipline. These were the changes that benefitted surgery.

For there could have been a very different outcome, if the unplanned and unforeseeable transfers of knowledge that did take place through different times and cultures, had not proceeded, or had fallen out of favour, or been ignored at any stage through which the knowledge of the ancients actually passed, we would be intellectually poorer today.

So, this fourth period ended with a growing dissatisfaction with the progress of medicine as demonstrated by therapeutic nihilism that started in Poland.[54] This state of mind was soon to be changed as the supremacy of the Ancients finally faded into the background and was eclipsed by what was to follow and yet their operations are still practised to this day.

References:

1. Chapter 2. 1163 AD. Edict of Tours.
2. Constitutions of Clarendon: Council of Tours 1163. Conclarendon.blogpost.
3. *Ibid.* 1905, p 22–23.
4. *The Historical Relations of Medicine and Surgery to the End of the Sixteenth Century.* By T. Clifford Allbutt. Macmillan and Co, New York. 1905, T Clifford Allbutt. p 23.
5. *The Annals of the Barber Surgeons of London.* By Sidney Young. Blades, East and Blades. Abchurch Lane, London 1890. Reprint, forgottenbooks.com ISBN 978-1-332-86964-0, 2019, p 1.
6. *Ibid.* 2019, p 51–52. Guild of Surgeons.
7. *Ibid.* 2019, p 55–58. Company of Barber Surgeons.
8. *Certaine Vvorkes of Chirurgerie.* By Thomas Gale. Hall Rowland D. 1563. Boston Medical Library. Nabu public domain reprints.
9. *A History of Surgery. By Harold Ellis*. Greenwich Medical Media Ltd., London 2001. P 36–37. John of Arderne.
10. *Arabian Medicine and Its Influence on the Middle Ages.* By Dr Donald Campbell, Vol 1, 1926, p. 156. John of Arderne.
11. Chapter 2. c425 BC., Hippocrates.
12. Wikipedia. Giovanni da Vigo.
13. Wikipedia. 1585. Ambrose Paré.
14. *The Beginnings of Western Science.* David C Lindberg. University of Chicago Press. 1992. Copernicus, p 102–103.
15. *Andreas Vesalius, the Reformer of Anatomy.* By James, Moores Ball. Saint Louis, Medical Science Press, 1910. Trieste Publishing 2017 by Lightening Source, Milton Keynes, UK.
16. *Certaine Vvorks of Chirurgerie*, by Thomas Gale, 1507-1587. Hall, Rowland, D. 1563 Printer.
17. *Several Chirurgical Treatises.* By Richard Wiseman. Printed by R. Norton and F. Macock, for R. Royfton Bookfeller to His Moft Sacred Majesfty at the Ship in St. Pauls Church-yard. 1686. Early History of Medicine, Health and Disease. Reproduced in the Henry E. Huntington Library and Art Gallery. Microfilmed in 1989.

18. *The Annals of the Barber Surgeons of London. Compiled from the Records and other Sources by Sidney Young.* Printed by Blades, East and Blades, London, 1890. Reprint, forgottenbooks.com. Henry Blackey, p 8.
19. Chapter 2, c1650. Dr Pimpernell.
20. *A History of Surgery.* By Harold Ellis. Greenwich Medical media Ltd., London, 2001. William Cheselden, p 187.
21. Chapter 2. c1650s. Dr Garengeot.
22. *Masters of Medicine, John Hunter, Man of Science and Surgeon.* By Stephan Paget. Leopold Classic Library. Originally Printed by T. Fisher Unwin, London, 1872. General background to John Hunter.
23. *Hunterian Reminiscences, Being the Substance of a Course of Lectures on the Principles and Practice of Surgery Delivered by John Hunter in the Year 1785.* Transcribed by Mr James Parkinson. Printed by Sherwood, Gilbert and Piper, Paternoster Row, London, 1893. Reprinted by Nabu Public Domain Reprints. p 104–105.
24. *Masters of Medicine, John Hunter, Man of Science and Surgeon.* By Stephan Paget. Leopold Classic Library. Originally Printed by T. Fisher Unwin, London, 1872. p 171–172.
25. *Chapter, p 170.* Aetius of Amida
26. *Arabian Medicine. Vol. 1.* By Dr Donald Campbell. Kegan Paul, Trench, Trubner and Co. Ltd. Carter Lane, London. 1926, Rhazes, p 86.
27. *Certaine Wworkes of Chirurgerie.* By Thomas Gale. 1507–1587. Printer, Roland D. 1563. Now in Nabu Public Domain Reprints, p 3.
28. Chapter 2. c170 AD. Antyllus.
29. *John Hunter. The Hunterian Reminiscences, being the Substance of a Course of Lectures on the Principles and Practice of Surgery, delivered by John Hunter in the year 1785.* By John Parkinson. 1878. Printed by Sherwood Gilbert and Piper. Paternoster Row, London. Hunter's operations. See Box 11.6.
30. Chapter 2. 1785. Parotidectomy, John Hunter's original operation.
31. *John Hunter. The Hunterian Reminiscences, being the Substance of a Course of Lectures on the Principles and Practice of Surgery, delivered by John Hunter in the year 1785.* By John Parkinson. 1878. Printed by Sherwood Gilbert and Piper. Paternoster Row, Hunter's series of lectures.

32. *The History of Medicine. A Very Short Introduction.* By William Bynum. Oxford University Press. 2008. p 43–44.
33. *The Life of William Savory.* Edited and Privately Printed by Stuart Eagles. Reading, Berkshire in 1994.
34. *The History of the Royal College of Surgeons of England.* By Zachary Cope. Anthony Blond Ltd, London, 1959. p 2.
35. *The Historical Relations of Medicine and Surgery to the End of the Sixteenth Century.* By Thomas Clifford Allbutt. Address delivered at the St Louis Congress in 1904. Hard Press Publishing USA.
36. *The History of the Royal College of Surgeons of England.* By Zachary Cope. Anthony Blond Ltd, London, 1959. p 157–164.
37. Chapter 2. 1809. Dr Ephraim McDowell.
38. *The Cambridge Illustrated History of the World's Science.* By Colin A. Ronan. Book Club Associates, London. The Press Syndicate of the University of Cambridge. 1983, pp. 253–254. Robert Grosseteste.
39. *The Cambridge Illustrated History of the World's Science.* By Colin A. Ronan. Book Club Associates, London. The Press Syndicate of the University of Cambridge. 1983, p 255. Roger Bacon. And, *Medieval Philosophy: A Practical Guide to Roger Bacon.* By M. James Ziccardi, 2011, p 13.
40. *The Beginnings of Western Science. The European Scientific Tradition in Philosophical, Religious, and Institutional Context, 600 BC to AD 1450.* By David C. Lindberg. The University of Chicago Press, 1992, p 228. Albertus Magnus.
41. *The Beginnings of Western Science. The European Scientific Tradition in Philosophical, Religious, and Institutional Context, 600 BC to AD 1450.* By David C. Lindberg. The University of Chicago Press, 1992, p 232. St Thomas Aquinas,
42. *The Beginnings of Western Science, The European Scientific Tradition in Philosophical, Religious, and Institutional Context, 600 BC to 1450 AD.* by David C. Lindberg. University of Chicago Press. 1992. John Dunn Scottus, p 242.
43. Chapter 2. 1441. Printing Press.
44. Ibid. 1506. Foundation of Pathological Anatomy.
45. Ibid. Vesalius and Anatomy.
46. Ibid. Galileo Galilei.

47. Ibid. 1628. Dr William Harvey.
48. Ibid. 1665. Medical Journals.
49. Ibid. 1693. Identification of bacteria.
50. Ibid. 1799. The Hunterian Museum, London.
51. Ibid. 1846. Ether.
52. Ibid. 1846. Washing of hands.
53. Aristotle. A.E. Taylor. Dover Edition first published in 1955 in an abridged reprinting of the revised edition of 1919. ISBN 10: 0-486-20280-8. p 57, 58.
54. Chapter 2. Early 1840. Therapeutic nihilism.

Chapter 12: Fifth Period

1846 to 1981. Surgery in Modern Western Europe and the USA

Original Operations in the Fifth Period of Surgery in Western Europe and the United States of America with Subsequent Developments

1846. USA. Ether as a general anaesthetic and the beginning of modern surgery.

The introduction of General Anaesthesia was the most important development in the history of modern surgery. It ushered in this fifth and final period of planned elective surgery on the brain, in the thorax and in the abdomen. All the original operation that followed its introduction are presented in this chapter. It also stimulated and enabled revisions and improvements to the original operations in the first, second and fourth periods. At the end of this period, in 1981, all the organs and tissues of the body had been operated on and excised where possible.

The practice of anaesthesia began with Dr Crawford Williamson Long[1] (1815–1878) from Georgia in the USA, who was the first to use the inhalation of sulphuric ether as a general anaesthetic on the 30th March 1842. This was to remove a tumour from the neck of a patient. The anaesthetic was administered to Mr James M. Venable by his inhaling it from a towel. Unfortunately, Long did not publish this until 1849.

For on the 16 of October 1846, ether was again used as an anaesthetic to extract a patient's tooth without pain by Dr William Thomas Morton[2] (1819–1868). This was the first public demonstration of its use. Two weeks later, Morton successfully anaesthetised a patient for amputation of a leg at the Massachusetts General Hospital in Boston, USA. The news spread rapidly and Morton became famous with his name forever coupled with the use of ether. The technique spread so fast that within eight weeks Dr Francis Boott (1792–1863) anaesthetised a patient for a tooth extraction in London. Chloroform was first introduced and used as a general anaesthetic in 1847 by Sir James Young Simpson[3] (1811–1870) a Scottish obstetrician.

Associated improvements included intubation of the trachea took place from 1919. Nasal intubation of the trachea was developed by Sir Ivan Whiteside Magill[4] (1888–1986) an Irish anaesthetist in Mr Harold Gillies department of plastic surgery. The nasal route of intubating the trachea gave surgeons unobstructed access when operating in the mouth.

In 1942, muscle relaxants were introduced by Professor Harold Randall Griffith[5] (1894–1985), an anaesthetist in Montreal who used curare on a young man undergoing appendicectomy. For the first time, it was now possible to produce complete muscle relaxation in a patient under general anaesthesia. This greatly improved surgeon's ability to operate within the abdomen without a struggle against the powerful muscle spasm of the abdominal wall.

In 1967, the author while assisting at abdominal operations as a student at St Thomas's Hospital in London, observed what happened when the muscle relaxant wore off before the completion of an operation. The abdominal muscles went rigid with spasm, immediately causing the bowels to be forcibly extruded through the open abdominal incision. This made closure of the abdomen extremely difficult. The anaesthetists were wary of administering a further dose of muscle relaxant as calibration was difficult at that time and the likelihood of having to ventilate the patient after the operation was to be avoided. A few days later, the wound ruptured and burst open with the bowels again extruding out of the wound. The abdominal wall then had to be re-sutured under a further anaesthetic. This was an active demonstration of the difference that muscle relaxants made to operating safely within the abdomen.[6]

By 1946, patients undergoing an operation requiring anaesthesia were administered the triad of narcosis, analgesia and muscle relaxation, which is still used today. However, it took some years for safe usage of these drugs to be established due to the initial difficulty of calibrating them.

The means of abolishing pain during an operation has been sought since earliest times. In Peru, chewing coco leaves may have been helpful. The Ancient Greeks were familiar with henbane and hemlock and also grew opium poppies, from about 1,200 BC. Gourds containing opium from Greece[7] dating from this time have been excavated in Egypt.

An earlier attempt at general anaesthesia was by Hugh of Lucca who introduced a 'Soporific sponge' in about 1250. Its use and preparation were described by his pupil Theodoric[8] (1206–1296). 'Take opium and unripe juice of mulberry, of hyoscyamus, of the juice of the leaves of mandragora, juice of the wood ivy, of the seeds of lettuce, burdock, and water hemlock each one ounce (28.35 grams); mix together in a brazen vessel and place in it a new sponge and let the whole boil as long as the sun on dog days, until the sponge consumes it all. When needed place the sponge in warm water for an hour and let it be applied to the nostrils, until he who is to be operated on is asleep. When finished, in order to rouse him, place another sponge dipped in vinegar frequently to his nose and let the juice of fenugreek be squirted into his nostril. Presently, he awakes'. These attempts at anaesthesia were not successful enough to have stood the test of time. Without pure ingredients, accurate measurements or appropriate tests, the results must have been haphazard and sometimes fatal. What if Theodoric could have accurately calibrated the ingredients!

References:

1. Wikipedia, Crawford Williamson Long.
2. *A History of Surgery.* By Harold Ellis. Greenwich Medical Media Ltd. 2001 ISBN 1 84110 023 4, p 81.
3. *The Cambridge Illustrated History of Medicine*. Edited by Roy Porter. Publisher, the Press Syndicate of the University of Cambridge, 1996, p 229.
4. *A History of Surgery.* By Harold Ellis. Greenwich Medical Media Ltd. 2001 ISBN 1 84110 023 4, p. 145.
5. Gillies D.M.M., Wynands J.E: Obituary: Dr Harold Griffith 1894–1985. Can J Anes. 1985: 32: 580–2.
6. Author. Personal observation.
7. A prelude to ether anaesthesia, William W. Ford. New England Journal of Medicine. Vol. 231. Aug. 1944 No. 6.
8. *Theodoric of Lucca. Timeline History of Anaesthesia Society.* www.histansocorg.uk. timeline.

1846. Austria. Hand washing becomes mandatory before examining a patient.

Professor Ignaz Semmelweis (1818–1865) of Vienna, noted that the maternity ward, where he and his staff attended women in childbirth immediately following a session in the post-mortem room had a mortality of 18% among the mothers. While, the midwives, who had their own maternity ward in the same hospital had a mortality of 2%. Semmelweis recognised the unfavourable connection between a post mortem room and the maternity ward and laid down a regime of rigorous hand scrubbing, using soap and then dipping the hands into chlorinated water before he or his students attended a childbirth. Maternal mortality immediately fell to 1%, despite the fact that the cause of puerperal fever was unknown. It was not until 14 years later that the Germ theory of disease was established.[1]

Reference:

A History of Surgery. By Harold Ellis. Published by Greenwich Medical Media Ltd 2001.

1853. USA. Abdominal Hysterectomy.

This was the first major and original operation to be undertaken following the introduction of anaesthesia. When Dr Ellis Burnham from Lowell, Massachusetts carried out the first successful abdominal hysterectomy in 1853[1]. He then performed a further 15 hysterectomies of which only three survived. By 1900, the mortality following hysterectomy for fibroids had fallen to 5% while total hysterectomy carried a mortality of 10%. The high mortality was due to postoperative sepsis and was considerably reduced following the introduction of Lister's antiseptic method of operating in 1867.[2]

The first laparoscopic hysterectomy was by Dr Harvey Reich in 1988. A survey of 511 laparoscopic total hysterectomies from 1990 to 2002, found that there were no deaths. Twenty-four of the patients were converted to an open operation, nineteen for pre-existing adhesions, two for haemorrhage, two for cystostomy and one for colonic perforation.[3]

Historically, in 120 AD, Soranus of Ephesus (b.98 AD) carried out the first recorded vaginal hysterectomy.[4]

References:

1. Hysterectomy: a historical perspective. By Sutton C. Baillieres. Clin Obstet Gynaecol. 1997 Mar; 11(1): 1–22.
2. *Science Medicine and History. Essays on the evolution of scientific thought and Medical Practice. Written in honour of Charles Singer. Volume Two.* Chapter by Zachary Cope on *'Seventy years of abdominal surgery'*. Published by Oxford University Press 1953. p 341.
3. Total laparoscopic hysterectomy: our five-year experience 1990–2002. Ochsner J. Spring 10(1): 8–12.
4. Chapter 2. c120 AD. Soranus.

1856. England. Publication of Gray's Anatomy.

In 1856, the first edition of '*Anatomy: Descriptive and Applied'* by Dr Henry Gray (1827–1861) and illustrated by Henry Vandyke Carter (1831–1898) was published. In later editions, the title was shortened to *Gray's Anatomy.* Gray was demonstrator, curator and lecturer of Anatomy at St George's Hospital at Hyde Park Corner, London and Henry Carter had been a demonstrator of Anatomy at St George's. This was the first illustrated book of whole-body anatomy. It has been steadily revised and improved through more than forty editions.

Reference:

Gray's Anatomy. 40th Edition. Anatomy. The Anatomical basis of Clinical Practice. Editor in Chief, Dr Susan Standring. Churchill Livingstone, Elsevier.

1858. France. Microorganisms discovered and germ theory of disease confirmed.

The 'miasma theory' that epidemic diseases were caused by poisonous vapour or mist was propounded by Galen (130–c200 AD) and prevailed until disproved by Professor Louis Pasteur (1822–1895) in 1858.

A theoretical germ theory of disease had first been proposed by Girolamo Fracastoro (c1476–1553) in 1546. This remained unproven and was ignored leaving Galen's theory undisturbed.

It was Professor Louis Pasteur who disproved the doctrine of spontaneous generation. In a paper published in 1858, he demonstrated that yeast was responsible for anaerobic fermentation of sugar into alcohol and that contamination by airborne micro-organisms was responsible for fermenting beer and wine and also for turning milk sour. In 1862, he devised a process, named after him as 'Pasteurisation', in which heating contaminated liquids killed most microorganisms, proving his germ theory of disease. This led to the discovery of bacteria, protista (other single celled organisms), fungi, viruses and separately prions. It was Pasteur's careful experiments that finally put an end to the doctrine of spontaneous generation of micro-organisms.[1]

Koch's 'postulates' for identifying the microorganism that caused particular diseases followed in the 1870s.

Reference:

The Cambridge Illustrated History of Medicine. Edited by Roy Porter. Cambridge University Press. 1996

1860. Switzerland. Total thyroidectomy.

The accolade for the first total thyroidectomy, without inadvertently excising all the parathyroid glands at the same time, goes to Professor Theodor Kocher (1841–1917), who was from the age of thirty-one Professor of surgery at Berne University. He proceeded to carry out over 5000 thyroidectomies for gross goitres due to hypothyroidism, an endemic condition in Switzerland, due to low dietary iodine. He was awarded a Nobel Prize in 1909, the first surgeon to be so honoured.[1]

Looking to the past, Aulus Cornelius Celsus (c25 BC–c50 AD) was the first to describe a partial thyroidectomy.[2] Over 100 years later, Galen of Pergamon (130–c200 AD) described two cases of thyroidectomy in which the surgeon had injured one of the recurrent laryngeal nerves causing a weakening of the patient's voice. Galen was well qualified to recognise this complication of thyroid surgery. For he had been the first to identify the function of the recurrent laryngeal nerves when carrying out vivisection on pigs in Alexandria in Egypt. The effect of dividing these nerves on both sides of the neck in a pig had resulted in it being unable to make any sound.[3]

In the tenth century AD, there was a successful partial thyroidectomy in Moorish Spain by Ali Ibn Abbas (f 952), who was also known as Albucasis.[4]

Until 1860, partial thyroidectomy had been reserved for the worst cases of people with very large hypothyroid goitres that were causing difficulties breathing, due to compression of the trachea. The enlargement was due to iodine deficiency common in Central Europe. Professor Theodor Billroth (1829–1894) undertook these thyroidectomies in Zurich; his initial mortality was 40% mainly due to post-operative sepsis. Billroth then stopped operating on these patients and did not resume until the antiseptic technique of surgery had been introduced by Joseph Lister (1827–1912) in 1865. The French Academy of Medicine was also concerned by the high mortality and advised against further thyroidectomies.[5]

It was only in 1852 that a parathyroid gland, situated in intimate contact with the thyroid, was first identified. This was discovered in a rhinoceros by Professor Richard Owen (1804–1892). Owen was at that time the Hunterian Professor and Conservator of the Museum of the Royal College of Surgeons of England. The actual function of the parathyroid glands in controlling calcium metabolism was not established until the twentieth century.[6] It was then recognised that that the four parathyroid glands in humans could be excised inadvertently when carrying out a thyroidectomy and that this had added considerably to postoperative morbidity and mortality as a result.

The first thyroidectomy for hyperthyroidism was by Dr Charles Mayo (1865–1939) in Rochester, Minnesota in 1890. At about the same time, Dr George Crile (1864–1943) founder of the Cleveland Clinic in Ohio, USA, recognised that the high mortality following surgery in thyrotoxic patients was due to a 'thyroxine storm' caused by fatal amounts of thyroxine being rapidly released into the blood stream. Crile found that by heavily sedating his patients for several days before operating that this catastrophe could be avoided. Later, potassium iodide was given to patients for several days before an operation, reducing the operative mortality to 1%. In modern times, thyrotoxic patients are given 'carbimazole' for several days preoperatively to suppress the release of excess thyroxine at operation. This has been so successful that there have not been any further deaths from post-operative thyroid storms.

Radioiodine was first used experimentally in the treatment of hyperthyroidism in 1942. It became widely available for treatment in the USA[7] by the 1980s. Surgery remains a treatment for hyperthyroidism involving the whole gland, as it is also the option of choice for patients who do not wish to undergo radioactive iodine injection treatment due to their fear of irradiation. This fear which was genuinely strong, but unwarranted, was common in the 1980s and 1990s.[8]

Thyroidectomy still remains the treatment of choice for nodular goitres and some carcinomas.

References:

1. *A History of Surgery.* By Harold Ellis. Published by Greenwich Medical Media Ltd 2001.
2. Chapter 2. c180 AD. Celsus.
3. *Science Medicine and History. Essays in Honour of Charles Singer. Vol.I.* Oxford University Press. 1956. p 211. Galen on Anatomical procedures.
4. A review of the history of the thyroid. Saurav Sarker *et al.,* Indian Journal of Surgery. Feb. 2016. 78(1): 32–36.
5. The History of Thyroidectomy by A.E.B. Giddings. J R Soc Med. 1998;91: (Suppl. 33) 3–6.
6. *Science, Medicine and History, essays of the evolution of scientific thought and medical practice, written in honour of Charles Singer.* London. Oxford University Press Vol. 2. Editor E. Ashworth Underwood. *Richard Owen and the discovery of the parathyroid glands: 1953.* By Cave A.G.E, p 217–222.
7. Radioiodine and the treatment of hyperthyroidism: the early history. Swain CT and Becker DV. Thyroid. Pub Med NCBI. 1998 Apr; 7(2): 163–176.
8. *The End of the Golden age of General surgery. 1870–2000.* By N.K. Maybury. CreateSpace Independent Publishing Platform, North Charleston, South Carolina. p 135.

1860. England. Foundation of the School for Nurses at St Thomas's Hospital, London.

In 1860, the Nightingale Home and Training School for Nurses at St Thomas' Hospital in London was opened by Miss Florence Nightingale (1820–

1910). It was the first to teach the precepts of modern nursing. Many of the nurses she trained rose to positions of authority not only in the major hospitals of Great Britain but also in the United States of America and the British Dominions and Colonies of that time.[1]

From an early age, Nightingale had been determined to do something to help other people and decided on nursing. This was then considered a low and dissolute profession and her parents would not allow it. Instead, she used her time to read the histories of hospitals and reports of medical commissions. On family holidays in Europe, she deserted the family group to visit hospitals and even worked at a nursing institution in Germany for three months. Once back in England, she applied for and became the Superintendent of a nursing home in Harley Street in London.

Following the outbreak of the Crimean War in 1854, Nightingale was appointed as Matron to the military hospital at Scutari near Istanbul. She brought 38 nurses with her and a considerable quantity of supplies that she had paid for herself. On arrival, she found the wounded from the battles were in a filthy condition, the food was disgusting and there was no linen or even cutlery. The smell of sewage and suppurating wounds was overpowering. Working day and night, she revolutionised the nursing and gradually brought order and cleanliness to the wards. From then on, the wounded had regularly washed sheets and clothes together with better food with cutlery.[2] For her late-night ward-rounds, she became known as the, 'Lady of the Lamp'.

On returning to England, Nightingale was extremely popular due to her success in Scutari. This, together with her nursing experience, considerable administrative skills, a forceful personality and sheer hard work enabled her to persuade government to appoint a Royal Commission to look into all aspects of military medical care. She was not only a nurse but also an able administrator and the foremost expert on sanitation and hospital building.[3]

References:

1. British library entry for a book in the Wellcome Collection https://www.bl.uk/collection-items/the-nightingale-home-and-training-school-for-nurses-st-thomass-hospital.
2. Wikipedia Florence Nightingale.

3. *Eminent Victorians.* The Biography of Florence Nightingale by Lytton Strachey. Chatto and Windus, 1918.

1865. England. Introduction of the antiseptic surgical technique that reduced wound infection.

From antiquity, the greatest cause of post-operative death was sepsis. Professor Joseph Lister (1828–1912) was aware of Professor Louis Pasteur's work that germs were the cause of sepsis. This stimulated him to develop a method of using carbolic acid as an antiseptic while patients were undergoing amputation of a limb, complicated by a compound fracture. A compound fracture is by definition an injury in which the skin as well as other tissues are penetrated by broken bone, enabling pathogenic organisms to enter and cause infection and sepsis. His technique was to spray carbolic acid on the instruments, dressings and the wound throughout the operation to kill bacteria. He also insisted on hand washing and clean surgical garments.[1] His technique was quickly accepted in Denmark and Germany where in 1875, he was given a warm welcome;[2] however, it took longer to be accepted in the United Kingdom and the United States of America.

In 1876, Lister was the chairman of the Surgical Section at a meeting of an International Surgical Congress in Philadelphia. At the end of two days' discussion, he was mortified when the meeting voted that they could not come to any distinct conclusions concerning the usefulness of his antiseptic method. Despite this, his advocacy of it was gradually accepted and used more frequently during the next few decades.[2]

The effectiveness of carbolic acid in preventing sepsis was demonstrated in 1876 by Sir William Macewen (1848–1924) a pupil of Lister's. Macewen, when Regius Professor of Surgery at Glasgow University later presented a series of 1,800 osteotomies without a single death caused by sepsis.

Soon afterwards in 1879, Sir Robert Lawson Tait(1845–1879) of the Birmingham Hospital in England moved away from the antiseptic technique devised by Lister. He developed an aseptic technique of operating to replace it. This resulted in surgical operations being conducted with scrubbed hands, sterile gloves, sterilised instruments and drapes. This new technique was quickly accepted and replaced the antiseptic method to become the worldwide standard for sterilisation and cleanliness during operations to this day.[3] Sepsis, the greatest cause of post-operative mortality and morbidity, was at last coming under control.

References:

1. *Science Medicine and History. Essays on the evolution of scientific thought and Medical Practice.* Written in honour of Charles Singer. Volume Two. Chapter by Zachary Cope on *'Seventy years of abdominal surgery'.* Published by Oxford University Press 1953, p 342.
2. *Sir D'Arcy Power, A Short History of Surgery.* London 1933.
3. Wikipedia. Sir Robert Lawson Tait

1867. France. First Splenectomy.

Dr Jules-Emile Pean (1830–1898) at St Louis' Hospital in Paris operated on a young woman for what had been diagnosed preoperatively as an ovarian tumour. The operation revealed an enormous splenic cyst that was successfully removed with the spleen.

The first successful splenectomy undertaken as an emergency operation following blunt trauma was by Dr Oskar Rienger (1844–1910), Surgeon at All Saints Hospital in Breslau in 1893. The first time that a delayed rupture of the spleen was recognised and operated on was by Sir Charles Alfred Balance (1865–1936) at St Thomas's Hospital, London in 1895.[1]

Total splenectomy then continued as the operation of choice for all splenic trauma resulting in haemorrhage until the early 1980s. This was when a detailed re-examination of the anatomy of the spleen showed each segment was served by a single artery. This made it possible for the surgeon to excise the damaged segments, while preserving the rest of the spleen. The confidence to carry out this operation was boosted by technology in the form of an ultrasound scan that could identify internal post-operative haemorrhage that might then be treated by aspiration rather than another operation.[2]

References:

1. *A History of Surgery.* By Harold Ellis. Greenwich Medical Media Ltd. 2001.

2. *The End of the Golden Age of General Surgery 1870–2000. The training and practice of a general surgeon in the late twentieth century.* By N. K. Maybury. Amazon Independent Publishing Platform. ISBN 1499531370. 2014. p 102–104.

1869. Germany. First elective nephrectomy.

A planned nephrectomy was carried out by Dr Gustav Simon (1824–1876) in Heidelberg in 1869. His patient was a woman who 18 months earlier had a segment of the left ureter excised while undergoing the removal of an ovary, resulting in multiple fistulae discharging urine. Simon decided that the only treatment was to remove the kidney. To perfect his technique, he operated on 30 dogs. His dogs and his patient survived.[1]

Up until 1876, fourteen nephrectomies were carried out in England, only six of whom survived. In at least four of these cases, the preoperative diagnosis was of an ovarian cyst.[2] In 1877, a partial nephrectomy for renal carcinoma was carried out by Professor Vincenz Czerny. (1842–1916) Professor of Surgery at Heidelberg, Germany.

The first nephro-lithotomy, the removal of kidney stones, was performed in 1870 by Sir Henry Morris (1884–1926). The diagnosis of the presence of stones in the patient's kidney was made entirely from the history and the clinical examination, for the 'stones' were easily palpable.

References:

1. *A History of Surgery.* By Harold Ellis. Greenwich Medical Media Ltd. 2001.
2. *Science Medicine and History. Essays on the evolution of scientific thought and Medical Practice. Written in honour of Charles Singer. Volume Two.* Chapter by Zachary Cope on 'Seventy years of abdominal surgery'. Published by Oxford University Press 1953, p 341.

1871. England. Operative treatment for ileo-caecal intussusception in children.

Intussusception, where the terminal ileum invaginates into the caecum, was first successfully reduced at laparotomy in 1871. This was by Mr Jonathon Hutchinson (1828–1913) of the London Hospital. Before this operation, intussusception was usually fatal. Hutchinson had previously published a review of 131 post mortem case reports dating back to 1847. As a result, he urged that this condition should be treated by surgery. Professor Harold Ellis, in his *History of Surgery,* was touched when reading the post-mortem report and said it made 'sad reading indeed'. For the demonstrable simplicity of reducing most intussusceptions at laparotomy, popularised this operation with gratifying results for child, parents and surgeon.[1] To be recognised, it is only essential that the surgeon considers this condition when examining a child with pain on the right side of the abdomen. The diagnosis was confirmed by Barium enema and occasionally the pressure of the enema alone reduced the intussusception, but usually surgery is needed.

In 1899, Sir Frederick Treves (1853–1923) at the London Hospital listed other causes of intestinal obstruction. He was pessimistic and thought that, 'Operations on dehydrated and toxic patients were unsuccessful due to the patient's late presentation',[2] for at that time, there was no means to successfully rehydrate a patient. Adults with intestinal obstruction from any cause not involving an external hernia were not then offered surgery and died on medical wards.

Dehydration began to be correctable after 1899, but was not routine until the 1920s when a bronze cannula was inserted into a vein. This was not as simple as sliding a modern cannula into a vein. For it required a surgical incision through the skin and into a vein, usually the long saphenous vein at the ankle, where the cannula was tied in place. The vein soon

thrombosed and due to the cut down and ligature, the vein was thereafter unusable. The modern cannula was developed in the late 1960s and has been improved ever since. The technique of using a bronze cannula was first used during the Great War of 1914 to 1918 for the first transfusions of blood by Sir Geoffrey Keynes.[3]

Suitable saline and glucose solutions used to correct dehydration caused by vomiting or obstruction of the gut became available in 1923.[4] From the 1950s, surgeons routinely undertook the care of patients with bowel obstruction by correcting the dehydration before operating, with the result that most patients survived this previously fatal condition. By the end of the 20th century, patients were coming to hospital earlier in the disease process with an improved rate of survival.

References:

1. *A History of Surgery.* By Harold Ellis. Greenwich Medical Media Limited, 2001.
2. & 4. *Seventy Years of Abdominal Surgery by Sir Zachary Cope. Science Medicine and History. Essays on the evolution of scientific thought and medical practice.* Volume Two. Oxford University Press 1953, p 341.
3. *Blood Transfusion.* By Geoffrey Keynes. Book published in 1923.
4. Chapter 2. 1902. Introduction of intravenous fluids.

1873. Austria. First laryngectomy for cancer.

In 1873, Professor Theodor Billroth (1829–1894) in Vienna carried out the first successful laryngectomy. The patient survived for seven months before dying from a recurrence of the tumour[1]. There was a possibility that a total laryngectomy might have been carried out in 1866 by Dr Henry H. Watson in Scotland.[2] This was not the case as the 'laryngectomy' was in fact a post-mortem excision of the larynx, that had been carried out on a patient who had died from syphilis.[3 & 4]

Until the 1980s, the only option for treating patients with established laryngeal cancer was excision of the laryngopharynx, along with half of the thyroid, with its associated parathyroid glands and an extensive dissection of the lymph nodes in the neck. These patients were left with a permanent tracheostomy. The survival at five years was 20%.[5]

Before 1873, all patients with cancer of the larynx died from the disease. Major surgery was then the only treatment, until the introduction of radiotherapy, chemotherapy and laser ablation of small tumours and the development and use of monoclonal antibodies. Antibody treatment was first introduced in 1986[6] and was tailored for each patient individually through genetic sequencing. This industry is now worth 20 billion dollars a year in the USA.[7] It is not beyond the imagination that if a cancer can be identified early enough surgery will become unnecessary and ultimately obsolete.[8]

References:

1. Dr Theodor Billroth and the first laryngectomy – NCBI. https://www.ncbi.nlm.nih.gov.pubmed
2. Total Laryngectomy – Past, Present, Future. Maedica (Buchar). 2014 Jun; 9(2): 210–218.
3. Laryngeal Syphilis: a case report. Arch Otolaryngeal Head Neck Surgery. 2011: Lahav G, Lahav Y, Ciobotaro P, *et al.,* 137; 294–298. (PubMed).
4. Transactions Internat. Med. Congress, vol. iii, 255.
5. *Bailey and Love's Short Practice of Surgery.* By A.J. Harding Rains and H. David Richie H.K. Pub. Lewis and Co. Ltd. London, 1987.
6. Biological Therapy Treatment, Laryngeal cancer. Cancer Research UK, 2018.
7. The History of monoclonal antibody development. Ann Med Surg (Lond). 2014 Dec; 3(4); 113–116.
8. *The Changing Face of Surgery.* An Inaugural Lecture by Professor Sir Peter Bell. Leicester University Press 1975.

1877. Germany. First esophagectomy.

Professor Theodor Billroth (1829–1894) in Vienna was the first to suggest the possibility of excising part of the oesophagus for malignant disease. Dr Vincenz Czerny (1842–1916) Professor of Surgery at Heidelberg and formerly a pupil of Billroth was the first to carry out an oesophago-gastrectomy. His patient died of a recurrence of the disease a year later. Sir Frederick Treves (1853–1923) in his 'Manual of Operative Surgery' published in 1910, considered the results of the operation to be very poor and doubted that the operation was ever justified.[1]

Indeed, the operation for excising a cancer of the oesophagus has not changed much since it was first devised. It is a major undertaking in two phases. The first is an upper abdominal operation to mobilise the stomach, so it can be drawn into the chest to replace the excised oesophagus. This wound is closed and the patient is then turned onto their left side so the right side of the chest can be opened through a thoracotomy and the cancer removed. The stomach is then drawn into the chest and joined to the remnant of the oesophagus[2] before closing the chest. Since the 1980s, treatment has also included chemotherapy and radiotherapy.

In the early twenty-first century, a trial to compare a laparoscopic operation with open surgery was undertaken. The laparoscopic approach reduced the post-operative complications and hospital stay, but did not alter the prognosis, as the disease is often advanced when diagnosed. Screening those at risk will be the only way to improve the five-year survival in the future. In the USA in 2015, 72% of patients who were diagnosed early, survived five years, this dropped to only 41%[3] in those with a late diagnosis.

References:

1. *A Manual of Operative Surgery,* Volume 1, by Frederick Treves. Published by Lea & Febiger. 1910.
2. *The Golden Age of General Surgery. 1870–2000. The training and practice of a general surgeon in the late 20th century.* By Nigel Keith Maybury. Publisher Amazon. ISBN 13: 9881499531374, 2014. p. 112–114.
3. Cancer.Net. 2005–2017 American Society of Clinical Oncology. Esophageal surgery.

1879. Scotland. First successful excision of an intracranial tumour, diagnosed preoperatively.

Sir William Macewen (1848–1924), Regius Professor of Surgery at Glasgow University, demonstrated that by clinical examination alone it was possible to indicate the side and site of an intracranial tumour. In 1879, he preoperatively diagnosed a tumour on the left side of the brain in a patient, localising it to the lower and middle portions of the ascending convolutions. At operation, this proved correct and he removed a large subdural tumour. Following the patient's death eight years later, an autopsy revealed no sign of a recurrence.[1]

Macewen was one of only two surgeons who undertook three original operations, the other was Theodor Billroth. Vascular brain tumours were very difficult to operate on due to severe haemorrhage. In 1926, diathermy was introduced enabling the surgeon to coagulate small blood vessels. This was successfully used by Dr Harvey Cushing (1869–1939), Surgeon-in-Chief at the

Peter Bent Brigham Hospital in Boston, USA. He was also a leader in the management of penetrating injuries of the brain in the First World War.[2]

Reference:

1. Wikipedia. Sir William Macewan
2. *A History of Surgery.* By Harold Ellis. Greenwich Medical Media Limited 2001.

1879. Germany. First cystoscopy with electric light.

On the 2nd of October 1877 cystoscopy with electrical illumination was demonstrated by Professor Max Nitze (1848–1906) in Berlin. He then worked with Joseph Leiter of Vienna, an instrument maker, who by October of 1879 had improved the instruments. The cystoscope revolutionised inspection and treatment of the bladder for stones and tumours.[1]

Reference:

1. *Seventy Years of Abdominal Surgery by Sir Zachary Cope. Science Medicine and History. Essays on the evolution of scientific thought and medical practice.* Volume Two. Oxford University Press 1953. p 341.

1879. Germany. First colectomy.

The first successful resection of a colonic cancer with end-to-end anastomosis was by Professor Vincenz Czerny (1842–1916) at Heidelberg in 1879. He was formerly an assistant to Professor Theodor Billroth. By 1899, Czerny's series of resections numbered 58 with a 37% mortality

mainly due to sepsis, usually peritonitis, caused by leakage or necrosis at the suture line on the colon. By 1895, a staged resection of a colonic carcinoma was developed. In the first stage, the tumour was exteriorised outside the abdomen. In the second, the tumour was resected and a double-barrelled colostomy formed. In the third stage, the double-barrelled colostomy was closed. Mortality was reduced to 12.5%.[1]

The need for a staged operation was also appropriate when the bowel was obstructed or had perforated. These patients were desperately ill and often presented at a late stage of the disease, this was still common 70 years later in the 1960s.[2] By then, the operation was reduced to two stages. The first being resection of the cancer with either a single or double-barrelled colostomy and the second being closure of the colostomy if that was possible. Following the introduction of plain x-rays and barium enema, a colonic cancer could be identified before it caused obstruction of the bowel. Under these circumstances, excision of the cancer and anastomosis of the bowel became possible in a single operation. By the 1980s, colonoscopy was the investigation of choice and had the advantage that biopsies could be taken at the same time to confirm the diagnosis.

In 1903, a sigmoid colectomy for acute diverticulitis was carried out by Professor James Rutherford Morrison (1853–1939), Professor of Surgery at Durham, England. This was principally a disease of the 20th century and is not mentioned in Sir Frederick Treves' 'Manual of Operative Surgery' published in 1892. Diverticulitis is associated with industrialisation, urbanisation and an ageing population living on a low residue diet. It is now increasing significantly in Asia and Africa. The disease still presents a problem in the USA, where there were over 300,000 admissions in 2009.[3]

References:

1. *A History of Surgery.* By Harold Ellis. Greenwich Medical Media Ltd. 2001.
2. *Seventy years of abdominal surgery by Sir Zachary Cope in Science and medicine in History. Essays on the Evolution of Scientific Thought and Medical Practice. Volume Two.* Edited by E. Ashworth Underwood. Oxford University Press, 1953. p 341.
3. Epidemiology and Pathophysiology of Diverticular Disease. M.R. Matrana and D.A. Margolin. Clin Colon Rectal Surg. 2009 Aug: 22(3): 141–146.

1881. Austria. First gastrectomy.

The first successful partial resection of the stomach for a carcinoma of the pylorus was by anastomosing the upper stomach remnant to the duodenum. This was carried out in 1871 by Professor Theodor Billroth (1829–1894) in Vienna. This operation became known as the 'Billroth 1 gastrectomy'.[1]

An earlier attempt to resect a tumour of the pylorus had been made by Dr Jules-Emile Pean (1830–1898) in Paris in 1879. The patient died on the 5th post-operative day. In 1870, a Polish surgeon Dr Ludwik Rydygier (1850–1920) at the University of Lwow carried out the same operation with the patient dying 12 hours postoperatively. Billroth knew of Pean's failure and had then worked out the technical details of the operation in an animal laboratory before he operated on a patient.[2] His patient survived and so fulfilled the criteria for his operation to be accepted as an original operation.

In 1898, a total-gastrectomy for cancer was carried out by Carl Schlatter (1864–1934) of Zurich, who following excision of the stomach, closed the duodenum and brought up a loop of jejunum to anastomose to the oesophagus. In 1969, a pouch fashioned from a portion of the upper jejunum was being attached to the oesophagus[3] to act as a reservoir to replace the stomach.

References:

1. Seventy Years of Abdominal Surgery by Sir Zachary Cope. *Science Medicine and History. Essays on the evolution of scientific thought and medical practice.* Volume Two. Oxford University Press 1953. p 341.
2. *A History of Surgery by Harold Ellis.* Greenwich Medical Media Ltd. 2001.
3. William Stewart Halstead. By Cameron J.L. Ann. Surgery. 1998; 225: 445–458.

1882. Germany. First cholecystectomy.

Dr Carl Langenbuch (1846–1901) was Chief of the Surgical Department at the Lazarus Hospital in Berlin, when on the 15th of July 1872, he carried out the first successful cholecystectomy on a 43-year-old man.[1] In the same year, Dr William S. Halsted (1852–1922) carried out a cholecystectomy at Johns Hopkins Hospital in Baltimore, USA.[2]

In 1879, gallstones obstructing a patient's common bile duct were removed at operation by Dr Robert Abbe (1851–1927) in New York and a few weeks later by Mr J Knowsley Thornton (1845–1904), in London.[3] The first acknowledged laparoscopic cholecystectomy was in 1985.[4]

In 1687, Dr Stal Von der Wiel, while draining an abscess in the right upper quadrant of a patient's abdomen found gallstones in the pus.[5] This was not considered an original operation, for this was a simple operation to drain an abscess and the gallbladder was not removed.

References:

1. *Seventy Years of Abdominal Surgery by Sir Zachary Cope. Science Medicine and History. Essays on the evolution of scientific thought and medical practice.* Volume Two. Oxford University Press 1953. p 341.
2. Wikipedia. Carl Langenbuch.
3. *A History of Surgery.* By Harold Ellis. Greenwich Medical Media Ltd. 2001.
4. Chapter 2. 1985. p 102.
5. Historical Perspective of Gall Stone Disease. Surg. Gynecol. Obs. 1984; 158: 81.

1883. England. Emergency salpingectomy due to ectopic pregnancy.

In 1883, Mr Robert Lawson Tait (1845–1889) of Birmingham, England, diagnosed preoperatively that a woman was suffering from a catastrophic intraperitoneal haemorrhage due to a ruptured ectopic pregnancy. An emergency operation was successful in saving her life. Tait became the leading authority in Europe on this condition. Before this a post-mortem study published in 1846 by Dr William Campbell,[1] looked into the causes of women dying unexpectedly during pregnancy. The commonest cause of death was found to be rupture of an ectopic pregnancy.

Ectopic pregnancy is caused by an ovum that has been fertilised abnormally in one of the fallopian tubes. This is usually associated with destruction of the cilia, the fine hair-like structures that normally propel the ovum to the uterus for fertilisation. The cause is usually due to a previous infection that damaged the cilia, so enabling sperm to enter the tube and fertilise the ovum there. It then becomes attached to the wall of the fallopian tube, instead of embedding itself in the lining of the uterus. Rapid embryonic growth within the narrow fallopian tube causes that structure to rupture and is accompanied by uncontrolled arterial bleeding into the peritoneal cavity. Due to the large space of the peritoneal cavity, the bleeding is not stopped as counter pressure cannot build up, resulting in exsanguination and death of the mother.

Tait recognised that this was a surgically curable condition, he also discovered that cases of fallopian pregnancy were not so rare as his colleagues asserted.[2] A few years later, a meeting of the Obstetrical Society of London expressed their collective opinion, 'That the great impediment (to treatment) was the uncertainty of diagnosis and no surgeon had yet performed a laparotomy for relief of this accident'.

Tait described death from this cause as the most 'dreadful calamity to which women can be subjected' and rejected the opinion of his colleagues. He set out to prove that an accurate diagnosis could be made from the history and physical examination. Between 1873 and 1878, he carried out 42 emergency operations[3] on women who had suffered an ectopic rupture. There were two deaths; in the first of these, he had not tied the artery supplying the fallopian tube. In the second, the patient died from shock due to blood loss. The fact that 40 women survived, all of whom would have otherwise died, attests to the skill and tenacity of Tait.[1]

Tait had proved that the correct diagnosis could be made from a careful history and examination when a pregnant woman presented with pain in the lower abdomen and showing the signs of shock. He told his colleagues, 'All that was needed was for the surgeon to think of the diagnosis'.

Now in the 21st century, a woman with a ruptured ectopic pregnancy is among the few emergencies for which an operating theatre will be opened at night.

Reference:

Lectures on Ectopic Pregnancy and Pelvic Haematocele. By Lawson Tait. Birmingham: The Journal Printing Works. 1878. Reprint by Leopold Classic Library 2017. p 3, 4, 45

1883. Scotland. First elective operations on the spine and spinal cord.

On the 9th of May 1883, Sir William Macewen (1848–1924), Regius Professor of Surgery at Glasgow, removed the laminae of the fifth, sixth and seventh dorsal vertebrae in a patient with complete paraplegia of two years duration. Correction of this angular deformity of the spine resulted in a complete recovery and many similar cases were subsequently treated successfully with only one death.[1] In 1887 Sir Victor Alexander Haden Horsley (1858–1916)[2] also treated a similar case.

A paper was read before the Royal Medical and Chirurgical Society by Mr Gowers and Mr Horsley, concerning a successful excision of a spinal cord tumour. This was described by Sir Frederick Treves in his *Manual of Operative Surgery* published in 1910, that in earlier times operating on the spine following a fracture had resulted in postoperative sepsis. This was already known by Macewen who followed the 'aseptic' technique of operating in a sterile environment. The post-operative mortality fell dramatically and this marked a new era in the prevention of wound infection and sepsis.[3]

The earliest description of a spinal cord injury is to be found in the Edwin Smith Papyrus from Ancient Egypt from about 1,700 BC. The following diagnosis is easily understood by a modern reader over 3,700 years later.

The unknown surgeon dictated to his scribe, 'If you examine a man having a dislocation in a vertebra of his neck, and should you find him unable to move his two arms and his two legs on account of it (and) urine drips from his member without his knowing it, (and) his two eyes are bloodshot: it is a dislocation of a vertebra of his neck extending to his backbone, which causes him to be unconscious of his two arms and two legs. You should say concerning him; a person having a dislocated vertebra of his neck while he is unconscious of his two legs and arms and his urine dribbles, (has) an ailment not to be treated'.[4] The physician could do nothing for this man and penalties for a physician when a patient died having undergone treatment could be harsh.[5]

References:

1. *A Manual of Operative Surgery Vol. 1.* By Frederick Treves FRCS. Published by Cassel and Company Ltd, Second Thousand. 1892. Sir William Macewen, 296.
2. *A Manuel of Operative Surgery. Vol. 1.* By Frederick Treves. Leigh and Febiger, 1910. Sir Victor Alexander Haden Horsley, 297.
3. History of Spinal Cord Medicine by I.M. Eltorai, M.D. www.demosmedical.com/media/wysiwyg/pdf/LinChapterOne.pdf.
4. *The Edwin Smith Surgical Papyrus. Published in Facsimile and Hieroglyphic Transliteration and Commentary.* Volume 1. By James

Henry Breasted. The University of Chicago Press 1980. Amazon Kindle Edition.
5. Wikipedia. Code of Hammurabi.

1886. Ireland. Excision of a pharyngeal pouch.

The first excision of a pharyngeal pouch was accomplished by Mr W.I. Wheeler in 1886 in Ireland. The condition had been described by Dr A. Ludlow in 1769. This was found during a post-mortem examination on a patient who had complained of dysphagia during his lifetime. The site of herniation is through Killian's dehiscence between the thyropharyngeal and cricopharyngeal fibres of the inferior constrictor muscle of the throat. The pouch when excised is a sac with an epithelial lining. It is most commonly found in the peoples of northern Europe and usually occur about the seventh decade of life with an incidence of two per 100,000 people per year.

Reference:

Pharyngeal Pouch (Zenker's diverticulum). M.A. Siddiq, S. Sood, D. Strachan. Post Graduate Medical Journal, Vol 77, Issue 910. Aug 2001.

1887. USA. First appendicectomy.

The first case of acute appendicitis, correctly diagnosed preoperatively and successfully excised was by Dr Thomas Morton (1835–1903) of Philadelphia in 1887.[1] American surgeons led the way in making an early diagnosis of acute appendicitis and operating on patients who presented with right iliac fossa pain and tenderness as an emergency. Seven years earlier in 1880, Mr Robert Lawson Tait (1845–1899), a surgeon in Birmingham, England, carried out a laparotomy on a right iliac fossa mass and found it was caused by a gangrenous appendix which he excised, this case was not published until 1890.

In general, the surgeons of Europe were slow to understand that acute appendicitis was a surgical emergency. One observer, an Australian surgeon Dr W.J.S. McKay[2] (d. 1948), wrote that he had never seen an appendix removed in any of the operating theatres in Europe when he visited twenty of the most celebrated clinics in 1892.

By 1900, removal of an inflamed appendix was becoming a standard procedure. Acute appendicitis is not without risk, for the famous poet, writer and

Nobel Laureate, Mr Joseph Rudyard Kipling (1865–1936) died following an appendicectomy at the Middlesex Hospital on the 18th of January 1936.[3]

References:

1. Paediatric Appendicectomy. Overview, Technique. Updated Nov 12 2015. Author: Mark V. Mazziotti. emedicine.medscape.com
2. *Seventy Years of Abdominal Surgery by Sir Zachary Cope. Science Medicine and History. Essays on the evolution of scientific thought and medical practice.* Volume Two. Oxford University Press 1953.3.
3. Wikipedia. Rudyard Kipling.

1889. England. First adrenalectomy.

The first successful adrenalectomy was in 1889 by Mr John Knowsley-Thornton (1804–1890), a London surgeon, who removed a 20-pound adrenal tumour along with the left kidney in a 36-year-old woman.[1]

The first planned adrenalectomy, through an abdominal incision was by Dr Perry Sargent in 1894. In 1927, Dr Charles Mayo (1865–1939) in the USA performed the first adrenalectomy through an incision in the flank. Over the next few years, both abdominal and flank approaches to excise the adrenal gland were made. The first laparoscopic excision of an adrenal gland was in 1992.

In 1941, Dr Charles Brenton Huggins[2] (1901–1998), Professor of Medicine at Chicago University, discovered that hormones could be used to control the spread of some cancers. He performed bilateral oophorectomies and adrenalectomies that were effective in controlling a third of cancers of the breast. In 1966, he was awarded a Nobel Prize. These operations became obsolete when chemotherapy was introduced.[3]

Historically, the first description and illustration of the adrenal glands was in 1552 by Bartholomeus Eustachius[4] (1520–1547) Professor of Medicine at the Collegio della Sapienza in Rome. If his research had not been lost, he might even have rivalled Vesalius as the father of modern anatomy.

References:

1. *Textbook of Endocrine Surgery*. By O. Clark, Q-Y. Duh, E. Kebebew. Elsevier, 2005.
2. Wikipedia. Charles Huggins.
3. *A History of Surgery*. By Harold Ellis. Pub. Greenwich Medical Media Ltd, London. 2001. P. 180.
4. *Andreas Vesalius, The Reformer of Anatomy*. By James Moores Ball. Published in 2007, Trieste Publishing Platform. P. 114–118.

1889. England. First excision of the pituitary gland.

The first transcranial hypophysectomy was carried out in 1889 by Sir Victor Alexander Haden Horsley (1858–1916), an eminent surgeon and Professor of Clinical Surgery at University College, London.[1]

In 1930, Harvey Cushing also used the transcranial approach, as some tumours were inaccessible from below. Post-operative sepsis was a dangerous and common complication resulting in a high mortality. The availability of antibiotics by the 1950s increased the success and safety of the operation.

In 1968, microsurgery was introduced for lesions visible radiologically.[2] Pituitary tumours that grow in size can cause visual-field disturbance, headaches and compression of the pituitary gland can cause hormonal deficiencies. Post-operatively hormone replacement medication is then necessary.[3] By 2011, pituitary tumours causing pressure symptoms were mainly operated on through the trans-sphenoidal route.[4]

References:

1. Wikipedia, Sir Victor Horsley.
2. Wikipedia, Stereotactic surgery.
3. *General Surgery Lecture Notes*. By Harold Ellis, Sir Roy Calne and Christopher Watson. Wiley-Blackwell 2011, p 108.
4. The evolution of trans-sphenoidal pituitary microsurgery. Wellbourn RB. Surgery. 01 Dec1986. 100(6): 1185–1190.

1892. England. First internal fixation of fractures.

In 1892, Sir Arbuthnot Lane[1] (1856–1943) of Guy's Hospital in London, found that setting fractures by manipulation and applying splints often led to an unsatisfactory result. In some cases, the bones did not unite resulting in arthritis of the neighbouring joints. Lane started to use wires and screws to stabilise fractures to achieve a better result. This required the exposure of the fracture surgically, converting a closed fracture into an open one, with a serious risk of introducing infection.

This operation was controversial when it was first carried out, as fifty percent of patients who had been treated by the generality of surgeons with metal implants died of sepsis. This was so serious that the matter was investigated by the British Medical Association. They ruled in Lane's favour, citing his meticulous adherence to Joseph Lister's antiseptic method of operating resulting in few post-operative infections. The investigation discovered that many other surgeons attempting to use the antiseptic method had lapsed in the detail and had thereby introduced sepsis into the wound. Lane also introduced steel plates to fix fractures in 1907.[1] In 1865, Lister used silver wire to fix a fractured patella.

In the modern era, open fractures continue to be fixed with screws and or plates and intermedullary nails or rods in fractures of the long bones. Wires are used in fingers and toes. All these innovations enable bones to heal and function sooner than otherwise would have happened.[2] These operations are dependent on antibiotic prophylaxis to prevent infection.

Reference:

1. Plarr's Lives of the Fellows, Royal College of Surgeons of England. Sir William Arbuthnot Lane.
2. Internal fixation of fractures from the American Academy of Orthopaedic Surgeons on line.

1892. Germany. First successful suture of a perforated Gastric ulcer.

An unsuccessful attempt to close a perforated gastric ulcer was made in 1887 by Mr J.W Taylor[1] of Birmingham. His patient died; it was of no comfort that this would have happened without the operation. By 1884, surgeons began to discuss whether patients with a perforated gastric or duodenal ulcer should be routinely offered surgery. They were encouraged by Billroth's success with the major operation of gastrectomy in 1881.[2]

On the 19th May 1892, the first successful operation to close a perforated gastric ulcer was by Dr Ludwig von Heusner of Barman (1843–1916). He operated at the patient's home where the light was bad and the operation so difficult that it took two and a half hours to carry out. It was however a success.[3]

In 1894, Mr Thomas Herbert Morse (1877–1921) of Norwich, England published a widely circulated report of a young patient he has successfully operated on for perforation. These successes established suturing perforated ulcers as an emergency procedure.[4]

References:

1. Seventy Years of Abdominal Surgery by Sir Zachary Cope. *Science Medicine and History. Essays on the Evolution of Scientific Thought and Medical Practice.* Volume Two. Oxford University Press 1953. p 341.
2. Chapter 2. 1881. Gastrectomy.
3. Wikipedia. Ludwig von Heusner.
4. Morse, Thomas Herbert. Biographical Entry in Plarr's Lives of the Fellows of the Royal College of Surgeons of England on line.

1894. England. First successful excision of an acoustic neuroma.

An acoustic neuroma was first identified at post mortem in 1777. The description described that, 'The neuroma was not firmly attached to the nerve but was fixed to the proximal part of the medulla oblongata at the point where the VIIIth cranial nerve makes its exit through the skull'.[1]

In 1890, an unsuccessful attempt to excise an acoustic neuroma took place with the death of the patient; it was an operation prone to serious complications, in particular haemorrhage and sepsis.

Sir Charles Alfred Balance (1856–1936) carried out the first successful excision of an acoustic neuroma in 1894. In 1917, Dr Harvey Cushing (1869–1939), an American Surgeon, devised a new surgical approach that solved many of these problems. Cushing's pupil, Sir Hugh William Bell Cairnes (1896–1952), who became the Foundation Nuffield Professor of Neurosurgery at Oxford, carried out the first total excision of an acoustic neuroma in 1931. The great breakthrough that enabled success with this operation was the development of technology, in this case the use of surgical operating microscopes.[2]

Surgery to excise an acoustic neuroma was an operation with a high mortality, and at the beginning of the 20th century, it was between 68–86% depending on the series. By 1960, it had been reduced to 10–20%. Now with early detection of small tumours being made by using a CT scan (computerised tomography) mortality has been reduced to 0.8%. The high mortality was initially due to the large size of the tumours due to late diagnosis, along with uncontrollable bleeding, herniation of the cortex, medullary compression and meningitis due to leakage of cerebro-spinal fluid followed by infection.

References:

1. History of the diagnosis and treatment of Acoustic Neuroma. Michael E. Glassock. Arch. Otolaryngol. 1968; 88(6): 588–585.
2. History of acoustic neuroma surgery. Theophilus G Machinis *et al.,* Department of Neurosurgery, Georgia. Neurosurg. Focus. 18(4): E 9. 2005.

1895. Scotland. First pneumonectomy.

The first successful pneumonectomy was by Sir William Macewen (1848–1924), Regius Professor of Surgery at Glasgow University, who carried out a total pneumonectomy of a tuberculous lung. The major technical problem of this operation was to prevent massive bleeding from the hilum of the lung, where the great pulmonary vessels are to be found. Macewen tied them all in a single ligature. The operative technique later metamorphosed to a careful dissection of the individual vessels, each being separately secured by ligation or suture. Macewen also made major contributions to the development of surgery in other fields including neurosurgery and orthopaedics, where he pioneered the use of bone grafts.

Reference:

History of Surgery by Harold Ellis. Greenwich Medical Media Ltd. 2001.

1895. Germany. The visualisation of internal organs. The Discovery of x-rays.

X-rays were discovered by Professor Wilhelm Conrad Roentgen (1845–1923), Professor of Physics at Wurzburg University, who presented his findings to the local medical society on the 28th December 1895. It was he who named them x-rays.

The first x-ray image of a human body part was of Roentgen's wife's hand. Within a month of the development of x-rays for clinical purposes, they were being carried out in Europe and the USA and within six months, they had become useful on the battlefield to locate bullets.[1] By 1896, chest x-rays were being taken in Scotland by Alan Campbell Swinton (1863–1930), a consulting electrical engineer and also in Boston Massachusetts, USA. Roentgen was awarded the Nobel Prize in Physics in 1901.

Reference:

Wikipedia. The discovery of X-rays.

1896. France. Discovery of radiation.

In 1896, Dr Antoine Henri Bequerel (1852–1908) a French physicist noticed that a small piece of uranium wrapped in paper and left on a photographic plate in a drawer for several weeks had left a mark on the plate when he developed it. The question was whether this was caused by another invisible ray?[1]

In 1898, Dr Marie Sklodowska-Curie (1867–1934), a graduate student at The University of Paris, undertook to investigate this phenomenon. Marie and Pierre Curie (1859–1906) on the 12th December 1898 discovered that a sample of uraninite consisted of two new elements.[2] By the end of the year, the Curies had identified them as polonium and radium.[3] In 1903, the Nobel Laureates for Physics were M. Henri Becquerel, Mme. Marie Sklodowska-Curie and M. Pierre Curie.

This seminal work led to the use of radiotherapy in the treatment of many cancers.

References:

1. *'Rayons emis par les composes de l'uranium et du thorium'.* Comptes Rendu, Vol 126, April 1898.
   Sur une nouvelle substance fortement radioactive, contenue dans le pitchblende.
2. . M.P. Curie, Mme. P. Curie *et al.,* M.G. Bemont, Comptes Rendu, Vol 127, Dec1898.
3. Henri Becquerel (1896). 'Sur les radiations emises par phosphorescence' Comptes Rendu. 122: 420–421, et 501–503.

1896. USA. First arterial reconstruction.

The first successful repair of an artery that had been severed by gunshot, was by Dr John Benjamin Murphy (1858–1916) of Chicago. He accomplished the anastomosis of this severed femoral artery by using a continuous suture. Murphy also performed and described modifications and improvements in neurosurgery, orthopaedics, gynaecology, urology, plastic surgery, thoracic surgery and vascular surgery.

References:

Wikipedia. John Benjamin Murphy.

1899. USA. Introduction of surgical gloves.

Rubber gloves were introduced by Dr William Halsted (1852–1922) at Johns Hopkins Hospital in Baltimore to protect the hands of the chief nurse in his operating theatre. She had developed a skin reaction to the corrosive properties of mercuric chloride then used as an antiseptic to prevent wound sepsis. Halstead rapidly implemented the general use of surgical gloves in the operating theatre. He also married the nurse.

The first disposable latex gloves were manufactured by Ansell in 1964.[1] These gloves became the cause of a serious clinical complication. The reason was that talcum powder had been used as a lubricant to make it easier for surgeons to pull the gloves on. This use of talcum powder led to a steady increase in the number of patients presenting as emergencies with distended abdomens caused by obstruction of the small bowel due to adhesive granulomas. The adhesions were an inflammatory reaction of the peritoneal lining of the abdominal cavity to talcum powder, causing loops of small bowel to stick together and stick to the lining of the peritoneal cavity. An alternative lubricant was then used and gradually, there was a decline in patients needing one or several sequential laparotomies to divide the intra-abdominal adhesions. This was a serious example of an iatrogenic, medically induced, complication.

Until the late 1960s, Casualty, now Accident and Emergency Department doctors did not routinely wear gloves when examining seriously injured or ill patients. Hepatitis B, C and aids were still in the future.[2] Now of course it is sensible as well as mandatory to wear gloves.

References:

1. Wikipedia. Latex surgical gloves.
2. Author. Personal note.

1899. England. Introduction of isotonic intra-venous fluids.

The earliest attempts to treat casualties with intra-venous fluids was in the Boer War in South Africa in 1899. Further attempts were made in the Balkan's War of 1912. The patho-physiology of electrolyte imbalance and hypovolaemic shock had been worked out by 1902. It was then possible for an isotonic saline solution to be prepared and used to replace blood and fluid losses during surgery. However, it was not until the end of the First World War that a cannula to deliver the fluid into a vein became available and improved the chances of a seriously dehydrated patient surviving.

Following the introduction of anaesthesia and the aseptic technique of operating, rehydrating a patient was the third most important factor in improving the survival of patients. This was only generally possible, following the development of modern cannulas in the 1960s, that could be inserted directly into a suitable vein, as earlier techniques had proved unsatisfactory. These included, injecting saline subcutaneously to replace fluid loss during an operation, as undertaken by Professor Oskar Reinger (1844–1910)[1] in 1893 and during World War One infusing saline into the rectum,[2] that also proved ineffective.

Sir William Brooke O'Shaughnessy FRS (1808–1889), a Scottish physician and chemical pathologist, examined the fluids and measured the specific gravity of the excreta of cholera victims. It was he who discovered the saline deficiency in the bloodstream and indicated the possibility of replacing it. He wrote that this would require injection of a saline solution into a vein.[3]

In the great cholera epidemic of 1832, Dr Thomas Aitchison Latta (1796–1833) was the first to treat a patient who was moribund and near the point of death due to dehydration. 'She was pale, her eyes were sunken, extremities cold and her jaw was dropped'. Latta inserted a tube into a vein and using a syringe repeatedly injected saline through it. After six pints of fluid, she revived and began to talk. Unfortunately, she did not survive. The results were published in the Lancet in 1832. Latta's technique was tried with enthusiasm on other cholera sufferers, but was abandoned, as the strength of the electrolyte content of the fluid to be injected could not then be measured. Few of these patients survived.[4]

Note.[5] Even in modern times, patients needing intravenous fluid hydration postoperatively must not be given only normal saline, as the kidneys cannot quickly excrete excessive sodium that has been infused. It results in severe oedema, heart failure and even death. Instead, a patient's daily sodium requirements need to be calculated and the correct amount of sodium infused in a balanced mixture of saline, dextrose or dextrose-saline. The author has included this note because when visiting a friend on the third day after a major abdominal operation in 2017, he noted that only normal saline had been infused during these three days and the patient was already grossly oedematous. After drawing attention to this, the intra-venous regime was changed, but it took three weeks before the oedema was finally reabsorbed.

References:

1. Wikipedia. Oscar Ringer.
2. 1968 Personal communication from Mr Robert Wallace Nevin TD. FRCS., (1907–1980), Consultant Surgeon, St Thomas's Hospital, London and Dean of the Medical School from 1957 to 1968.
3. Moon J.B. (1967). Sir William Brooke O'Shaughnessy: The foundations of fluid therapy and the Indian telegraph Service. New England Journal of Medicine. 276(5): 283–284.
4. Wikipedia. Thomas Aitchison Latta.

5. Author's note.

1903. France. Surgery for liver failure due to cirrhosis and portal vein hypertension.

Dr E. Vidal, a French Surgeon performed the first portocaval shunt[1] in 1903. This was to alleviate gross ascites in a patient who had previously suffered several severe gastrointestinal bleeds due to portal vein hypertension. The patient survived four months.

Previously, in 1877 portocaval shunts were carried out on a series of dogs by Dr Nikolai V. Eck (1849–1908), a Russian Army surgeon. Professor Ivan P. Pavlov (1849–1936), another Russian who was the most famous physiologist of the late 19th and early 20th century was aware of Eck's work. Pavlov in 1893 also carried out this operation in dogs. He diverted the blood in the portal-vein, carrying nutrition from the gut to the liver, by anastomosing it to the inferior vena cava, the great systemic vein returning circulating venous blood to the heart. He observed that this led to the dog developing encephalopathy, a severe disturbance of the brain.[2] The encephalopathy was caused by toxic substances absorbed from the gut that were now diverted and reached the brain without being detoxified by the liver. This significantly reduced the usefulness of the operation.

The origins of cirrhosis and its sequelae were worked out during the next few decades. Drs McIndoe and McMichael[3] showed during the 1930s, that enlargement of the spleen also occurred in patients with portal-hypertension. The term portal-hypertension had been coined in 1906 and was already associated with ascitic fluid in the abdomen and cirrhosis of the liver. This high pressure in the portal veins caused them to rupture and bleed profusely.

Sclerotherapy for bleeding oesophageal varices was introduced in 1939 by Drs C. Crafoord and P. Frenckner, who used a rigid oesophagoscope through which to inject and obliterate fragile and dilated veins. From the 1940s to the early 1980s, the standard treatment to stop torrential varicocele bleeding was oesophageal balloon tamponade. This caused serious complications with 15% of patients suffering from aspiration pneumonia, oesophageal ulceration and rupture of the oesophagus. If tamponade did not stop the bleeding, or worse as described, then emergency surgery was carried out to divide the dilated veins at the junction between the oesophagus and stomach.

By the mid-1980s, flexible endoscopy had become generally established and the effectiveness of sclerotherapy to stop bleeding varices was further enhanced when a twin-channelled endoscope was developed, enabling varices to be injected and/or ligated using rubber bands.

Surgical portal vein to systemic vein shunts were reintroduced by Alan O. Whipple (1881-1963) in 1945 as elective as well as emergency operations. They relieved the pressure in the portal vein system by diverting the blood into the inferior-vena-cava as previously described. This operation continued as the mainstay of treatment from the 1960s to the mid-1980s and was as expected often accompanied by post-operative encephalopathy. This treatment had an operative mortality of 30–50% and only 30% of patients survived a year.

By the late 1980s, surgery was being replaced by medical treatment following the introduction of Vasopressin and Telipressin. These drugs successfully reduced the pressure in the portal vein. TIPSS, 'Trans-jugular Intrahepatic Porto-systemic Shunts' were then introduced. In this medical intervention, a metal stent is introduced via the jugular vein into the liver under radiological control. From there it is guided to make an artificial connection between the hepatic vein and a branch of the portal vein, thereby effectively relieving the portal hypertension, without completely bypassing the detoxification process of the liver.

By 2010, pharmacological treatment with endoscopic and radiological stenting therapies were now the treatment of choice to prevent varicocele haemorrhage from the stomach or oesophagus. These techniques reduced the side effects and a higher rate of survival was achieved. Broad spectrum antibiotics also reduce the incidence of sepsis. Blood transfusion is withheld if a patient's haemoglobin is 9 g/dL or above as this tended to raise the portal pressure, it was only when the haemoglobin falls below 7 g/dL that a transfusion is given. Torrential gastric haemorrhage leading to rapid exsanguination now came under further scrutiny and results further improved when thrombin was introduced and used to obliterate the varicose veins in the stomach and oesophagus[4].

Modern treatment now includes twenty-four-hour-endoscopy-rotas for the rapid employment of tamponade equipment,[5] endoscopy and TIPSS. Mortality has fallen from 42% in 1981 to 6–12% in 2014. The result of this success has made emergency surgery such as oesophageal transection and portocaval shunts obsolete.

This is an example of how complex and hazardous surgery has been rendered obsolete and replaced by medical intervention and treatment. However, the ultimate treatment for end stage cirrhosis and portal hypertension is still surgical, and is a liver transplant, the first of which was carried out in 1963.[6]

References:

1. Vidal E. Traitment chirurgical des ascites. Presse Med. (1903); 11: 747–761.
2. *I.P. Pavlov. Selected Works.* Edited by S. Koshtoyants, Corresponding Member of the U.S.S.R. Academy of Sciences. Moscow 1955.
3. *Portal Hypertension Surgical Treatment: Evidence-Based and problem orientated.* Li, J.C, Henderson, J.M. 2001. ncbi.nim.nih.gov. NCBI Bookshelf.
4. Historical overview and review of current day treatment in the management of acute variceal haemorrhage. Neil Rajariya and Dhiraj Tripathi. World Gastroenterology. 2014 June 7: 20921): 6481–6494.
5. Balloon tamponade. Robert Sengstaken (b. 1923) Neurosurgeon, New York, and Arthur H. Blakemore (1898–1980), Colombia Presbyterian Medical Centre, New York.
6. 1963. First liver transplant.

1904. USA. First radical prostatectomy for cancer.

The first radical prostatectomy for carcinoma was carried out in 1904 by Dr Hugh Hampton Young (1870–1945) and Dr William Stewart Halstead (1852–1922) at the Johns Hopkins Hospital in Baltimore, where they performed an extracapsular perineal prostatectomy.[1]

In 1945, Mr Terrence Millin (1903–1980) Surgeon at the All Saints Hospital, London, published the first series of radical retropubic prostatectomies for carcinoma.[2]

In 1991, the first laparoscopic radical prostatectomy was carried out and in 2011, a DaVinci robot assisted laparoscopic prostatectomy was performed.[3]

References:

1. The History of prostatic cancer from the beginning to DaVinci, by Hatzinger M, Hubmann R, Moll F, Sohn M. US National Library of Medicine National Institutes of Health. Aktuelle Urol. 2012 Jul; 43(4): 228–230.
2. Millin T. Retropubic prostatectomy. A new extravesical technique. Lancet 1945; 249: 711.
3. 2000. Robot assisted surgery.

1906. USA. First repair of an aneurysm and subsequent developments.

The original operation of repairing an aneurysm was in 1906, when Dr Rudolf Matas (1860–1958) of New Orleans, repaired a popliteal aneurysm and later described the results in a series of 19 patients. Matas' technique was to pass a catheter the diameter of a normal popliteal artery to lie within the aneurysm. The redundant wall of the popliteal aneurysm was sewn together over the catheter to give a normal diameter of the artery remnant, thus maintaining the flow of blood into the lower leg. In 16 patients, the operation was successful, one patient died and two subsequently needed amputation[1]. By 1913, a saphenous vein from a patient's leg was harvested, then after reversing it to prevent the venous valves from preventing the flow of arterial blood; it was then used to replace the aneurysmal segment of artery.

An aortic aneurysm was first replaced by a homograft in 1951 by Dr Denton A. Cooley (1920–2016), Surgeon-in-chief at the Texas Heart Institute and Dr Michael E. Debakey (1908–2008). This operation required the harvesting and denaturing of a human aorta to be used as the homograft[2]. By the 1980s, Dacron and other synthetic grafts became available and were produced in different sizes. This resulted in surgeons being able to select a graft of the right calibre after having inspected the aorta.

In 1953, Dr Henry T. Bahnson (1920–2003) Professor of Surgery of the University of Pittsburgh School of Medicine is credited with the first successful repair of a ruptured aortic aneurysm with a synthetic graft.[3]

Then the first successful stenting of an aortic aneurysm was in Buenos Aires in 1990, by Professor Juan C Parodi.[4]

The stent was introduced via a femoral artery using a compressible graft with a metal component to replace the suture. This was the beginning of a less invasive but effective procedure. It is another example of an operation being gradually replaced by a procedure. One of the benefits of this has been to reduce the incidence of ruptured aortic aneurysms. The overall post-operative mortality was reduced from 7% with the open operation to 4% by using a stent.[5]

The first successful carotid endarterectomy was carried out by Dr Michael E. Debakey in Huston in 1953.Atheroma can particularly affect the bifurcation of the carotid artery where it branches into the internal and external carotid arteries. Atheroma can ulcerate and throw off emboli causing blindness or a stroke. The operation was to remove the atheromatous plaque and then widen the bifurcation of the carotid arteries with a patch from a vein. By 2011, carotid angioplasty was being carried out more frequently, replacing the necessity for carotid endarterectomy.[6]

References:

1. Rudolph Matas and the first endoaneurysmorrhaphy: *A Fine Account of this Operation. Historical*
2. *Vignettes in Vascular Surgery.* By Michael C. Trotter. Editor Norman M Rich. https://core.ac.uk.
3. Wikipedia. Michael Debakey.
4. 1953 Henry T. Bahnson. Ann. Surg. 2003 Apr: 237(4): 591–592
5. Endovascular revolution in the aorta: 25 Years of a Landmark Case. vascularnews.com 2016.
6. The End of the Golden Age of General Surgery. By N.K. Maybury. Printed by Amazon. ISBN: 1499531370. 2014. P. 175–176.
7. Michael E. Debakey. Vascular Specialist. Published 2012 by Mark S. Lesney. mdedge.com

1906. Moravia. First successful full-thickness corneal transplant.

Unsuccessful attempts at corneal transplantation date back to the 1800s. In 1906, Dr Eduard Zirm (1863–1944) the Chief of Ophthalmology at Olomouc in Moravia, carried out a successful bilateral corneal transplant. This was in a labourer aged 45 who had suffered severe lime burns and whose corneas were opaque and a white-grey in colour. The patient was able to return to work.

Reference:

The first successful full-thickness corneal transplant: a commentary on Eduard Zirm's landmark paper of 1906. Br J Opththalmol. 2006 Oct: 90(10): 1222–1223.

1907. England. First radical excision of a rectal cancer.

In 1907, Mr John Percy Lockhart-Mummery (1875–1958) of St Mark's Hospital, London, excised a rectal cancer in two stages with the aim of developing a radical, curative operation. He approached the rectum from above through a lower abdominal laparotomy incision and formed a colostomy in the left iliac fossa. At the same operation or after a delay of days, he then excised the anus, rectum and associated lymph nodes. In 1926, he published a series of two-hundred patients with a mortality of 3% and a cure rate of 50%.[1]

After 1907, Mr William Ernest Miles (1869–1947) operating in what is now the Royal Marsden Hospital in London, where he perfected the technique of a synchronous, combined abdomino-perineal excision of the rectum. This requires two surgeons to operate simultaneously, one on the abdomen and the other on the perineum and became the standard approach for this operation by the 1960s.[2]

By the 1990s, preoperative chemo and radiotherapy was considered the standard treatment for stage I and II rectal carcinomas before surgery. This gave a considerable reduction in the size of the tumour to be operated on and achieved complete eradication of the tumour in 25% of patients with these stages of the disease.[3] This represents the beginning of a move away from radical surgery to medical intervention.

Historically, Dr Jacques Lisfranc performed the first perineal resection for a case of rectal cancer in 1826 when he removed only a few centimetres of the distal rectum. In 1874, Professor Theodor Kocher (1841–1917) introduced a trans-sacral resection with coccygectomy. Dr Paul Kraske (1851–1930), a German surgeon, further extended this operation to gain wider access to the tumour from below. In all these cases, there was very little space within which to operate from below and it was impossible to carry out a radical excision of the cancer. Moreover, the patients were left with what was an uncontrolled perineal colostomy. Because these were non-curative and left the patient incontinent, they have not been considered successful and therefore not designated as original operations.

In summary, management of patients with cancer of the rectum has improved dramatically following the introduction of chemo-radiotherapy. The resulting shrinkage or even eradication of the tumour by adjuvant treatment reduces the complexity of the operation making it more amenable to a laparoscopic excision. Coupling this with the ongoing nationwide screening programme to identify cancers of the colon at an earlier stage of the disease[4] could lead to better results. If this trend continues, which is by no means certain, then ultimately medical treatment may become the normal first line of treatment and further reduce the role of surgery in the treatment of this disease.

References:

1. Two hundred cases of cancer of the rectum treated by perineal excision. J.P. Lockhart Mummery. British Journal of Surgery. Volume 14, Issue 53 July 1926, Pages 110–124.
2. Annals of Coloproctology 2012 Aug: 30(4): 165–174.
3. Preoperative versus postoperative chemoradiotherapy for rectal cancer by Sauer R, Becker H, Hohenberger W. *et al.,* N Engl J Med 351: 1731–1740, 2004.
4. *The End of the Golden Age of General Surgery, 1870–2000. The Training and Practice of a General Surgeon in the Late Twentieth Century.* By Nigel Keith Maybury. Pub. Amazon Independent Publishing Platform. ISBN 1499531370, 2014, p 114–120.

1907. France. Curative myotomy for infantile pyloric stenosis.

Pyloric stenosis in infants was first identified as a fatal condition, when recorded at autopsy in 1717 by a Dr Blair. This condition was also confirmed by Dr Harold Hirschsprung (1830-1916) at an autopsy in 1887. It is a non-malignant condition that has the appearance of a smooth tumour caused by enlargement of the circular muscle of the pylorus. If this muscle enlarges, it compresses the normal passage between the stomach and duodenum and can rapidly progress to prevent even liquids from passing through. Babies suffering from this condition, typically present at about six weeks of age. The pyloric enlargement is caused by a genetic mutation where a neuronal nitrous oxide gene is absent.[1]

An infant with projectile vomiting was first treated surgically by a pyloromyotomy in 1907 by Dr Pierre Fredet (1870–1946) surgeon at the Pitié-

Salpêtrière Hospital in Paris and this was the original operation. He left the mucosa intact and re-sutured the muscle. The operation was simplified in 1911 by Dr Conrad Ramstedt (1867–1963), a German military surgeon who also divided the thickened muscle at the pylorus without opening the mucosa but left the myotomy open. This operation is still named 'Ramstedt's operation'. Before this, babies died from this non-malignant condition.[2] The operation is now usually carried out laparoscopically. Results are excellent and mortality is extremely rare.[3]

References:

1. *Paediatric Hypertrophic Pyloric Stenosis: Background, Anatomy and Pathophysiology,* by M.S. Irish. Emedicine.medscape.com. Updated Jul 5 2018.
2. Wikipedia. History of Pyloromyotomy.
3. *General surgery Lecture Notes* by Harold Ellis, Sir Roy Calne and Christopher Watson. 12th Edition, Wiley Blackwell, 2011.

1908. Germany. Introduction of diathermy by electro-coagulation.

The word diathermy was coined by Dr Carl Franz Nagelschmitd[1] (1875–1952) who carried out extensive experiments on patients using diathermy and published a text book on the subject in 1913. Surgical diathermy is the successor of ancient red-hot cautery as described in the Edwin Smith Papyrus[2] of about 1,700 BC.

Diathermy involves a high frequency A.C. current that can be used either as a cutting tool or to coagulate small vessels to stop bleeding. It is still an essential instrument for surgeons.

References:

1. Wikipedia. Electrocautery.
2. Chapter 2. c1700 BC. Edwin Smith Papyrus.

1909. Germany. First pancreatico-duodenectomy.

The first successful pancreatico-duodenectomy was by Professor Walther Carl Eduard Kausch (1867–1928), Professor of Surgery in Berlin in 1909. He carried out a two-stage operation and implanted the remaining tail of the pancreas into the distal stump of the resected duodenum.

In 1940, Dr Alan Whipple (1881–1963) of the Columbia-Presbyterian Medical Centre, USA, performed the first one stage pancreato-duodenectomy. The mortality from these early operations was 21%. By 1980, this had been reduced considerably and is now less than 1%. However, only 10% of patients with pancreatic carcinoma come to surgery and the five-year survival rate is less than 8%.[1]

Reference:

1. History of pancreatico-duodenectomy: early misconceptions, initial milestones and the pioneers. Chandrakanth Are, Mashaal Dhir and
2. Lavanya Ravipati. HPB (Oxford). 21 Jun: 13(6): 377–384.

1910. Germany. Introduction of laparoscopy and laparoscopic surgery.

Laparoscopic surgery is a revolutionary and advanced new way to carry out already existing operations. Therefore, operations performed laparoscopically are not original operations and have not been described as such in this book. It represents a new and less traumatic technique than open operations for carrying out a wide range of surgery. This represents a classic improvement to an original operation undertaken by successor surgeons.

Laparoscopic operations were first carried out over 100 years ago and were used by gynaecologists for diagnostic purposes and minor operations. The technique was pioneered by Dr Georg Kelling[1] (1866–1945) of Dresden in 1902, when he performed laparoscopic surgery on dogs. In 1910, Dr Hans Christian Jacobaeus[2] (1879–1837) from Sweden used a cystoscope to internally examine the thorax and abdomen in patients. His procedures are considered to be the first diagnostic laparoscopy and thoracoscopic examinations.

The first laparoscopic cholecystectomy was carried out, in 1985, by Dr Erich Muhe[3] (1938–2005) of Boblingen in Germany, who was a gynaecologist. Initially his work was not accepted for publication. However, seven years later in 1992, he was awarded the German Surgical Society's Anniversary Award, having being cited as performing, 'One of the greatest achievements in medicine in modern history'.

A year later in 1987, Dr Philippe Mouret[4](1938–2008), a French gynaecologist at Lyon in France, also carried out a laparoscopic cholecystectomy. Dr Francois Dubois (1938–2005) of Paris, learning about this operation, immediately borrowed instruments from the gynaecologists and after animal trials carried out a laparoscopic cholecystectomy in 1987. He reported the results in the USA.

By 1988, new instruments were designed to enable the gallbladder to be excised using a laparoscopic approach. A decade later, this was the operation of choice for cholecystectomy on every continent.[5] Laparoscopic cholecystectomy is now usually a day case procedure and represents a significant technical advance that benefits patients by reducing post-operative pain due to the small incisions and shortening of the hospital stay. The time needed for convalescence postoperatively has also been considerably reduced and represents an improvement on open cholecystectomy.

References:

1. Wikipedia. Georg Kelling.
2. Wikipedia. Dr Hans Christian Jacobaeus.
3. Wikipedia. Erich Mühe. And. Mouret, Dubois and Perissat: The Laparoscopic breakthrough in Europe 1987–1988. JSLS. 1999 Apr-Jun: 3(2): 163–167.
4. Twenty years of Laparoscopic Cholecystectomy: Philippe Mouret. JSLE. 2008 Jan-Mar; 12(1): 109–111.
5. *The End of the Golden Age of General Surgery. 1870–2000.* By N.K. Maybury. Published by Amazon Publishing Platform. ISBN 1499531370, 2014, p. 110–111.

1912. Germany. Thymectomy.

The first thymectomy was carried out by Dr D.R. Sauerbruch[1]

in Berlin in 1912. It was to alleviate the symptoms of weakness caused by myasthenia gravis. The first detailed account of the operation was by Dr Alfred Blalock[2] (1899–1964) in 1936. Before that, an enlarged thymus had previously been recognised at autopsy in 1877.

Myasthenia gravis is a rare disease where the body's own immune system attacks the nerves carrying signals to the muscles. The original surgical approach to excise the thymus was by splitting the sternum. Later, a less traumatic approach through a midline incision in the neck was used. A minimally invasive approach now has the advantage of being carried out as a day case and avoids the complications that splitting the sternum can cause.[3]

References:

1. *Myasthenia Gravis and Myasthenic Syndromes*, in Walton Jed. Disorders of Voluntary Muscle. 4th E. Edinburgh. Churchill Livingstone. 1981, p. 582.
2. Alfred Blalock and thymectomy for myasthenia gravis. Annals of Thoracic Surgery. 1987 Mar. 43(3): 348–9.
3. Extended transcervical thymectomy: the ultimate minimally invasive approach. Joseph B. Shrager. Ann. Thorac Surg. 2010; 89; S2128–34.

1915. England. Blood transfusion in World War I.

Sir Geoffrey Langdon Keynes (1887–1982) Surgeon at St Bartholomew's Hospital, London and brother to Dr John Maynard Keynes (1883–1946) the famous economist, served with the British Expeditionary Force in France in 1915. He worked in a field hospital near the battle front and while there devised a 'blood flask' that he used to transfuse wounded soldiers who had suffered severe haemorrhage and who had not been expected to survive.[1] The results were gratifying. Transfusion of blood was only sporadically used in the early years of that war, but by the end, it was being taken from donors and citrated ready for use before major battles commenced. It often prevented shock if given early enough to the wounded.[2]

In 1917, the Americans joined the Allies and also set up transfusion units in the war zone.[3] This eventually led to civilian transfusion units being developed in both Europe and America. The Red Cross organised a register of blood donors and by 1939, citrated blood had a useful shelf life of two weeks. Refrigerated blood and dried plasma were also available. Sir Lionel Whitby[4] (1895–1956), a British haematologist, organised the Blood Transfusion Service and ensured that enough blood was available from the beginning of the Second World War, to treat both wounded soldiers and civilians.

References:

1. *Blood Transfusion* by Geoffrey Keynes. Published 1923.
2. Seventy Years of Abdominal Surgery by Sir Zachary Cope. *Science Medicine and History. Essays on the evolution of scientific thought and medical practice.* Volume Two. Oxford University Press 1953. p 341.
3. Combat Casualty Care and Surgical Progress. Ann. Surg. 2006 Jun: 243(6): 715–719.:
4. Wikipedia. Sir Lionel Whitby.

1915. England. Surgical treatment of abdominal wounds in times of war.

In 1915, Mr Owen Richards (1873–1949) a British surgeon working in Military Hospitals near the battle front, in World War 1, carried out laparotomies on patients with gunshot wounds and resected perforated small bowel with success.[1] He carried out these operations against military medical regulations.

This was so successful that between 1915 and 1917, 3520 abdominal operations were carried out by British surgeons with a mortality of 53%. Although this is high, it must be compared with the 100% mortality in the first year of the war when laparotomy was not performed. This led to a significant change in attitude, as emergency surgery for both the acute abdomen and war wounds involving the abdomen had been neglected for many years.

Previously, the view of many surgeons had been that operative treatment of abdominal wounds was not advisable under battlefront conditions, as wounds were often complicated by high velocity missiles and bacterial contamination. This was the norm in Belgium and Northern France at the beginning of World War I. Gas gangrene caused by Clostridium welchii was commonplace, as also was tetanus caused from spores of the bacteria Clostridium tetani. To minimise the development of gangrene, the most effective treatment for all wounds was to debride them, excise all dead tissue and remove all foreign bodies while leaving the wounds open to facilitate drainage.[2]

During World War II (1939–1945), casualty clearing stations were placed as close to the battlefront as possible. This enabled faster evacuation and evaluation of the wounded and provided first line treatment. This consisted of debriding and cleaning wounds, the immobilisation of fractured limbs and emergency surgery for abdominal, chest and head wounds. These actions reduced the mortality from abdominal wounds to 25% compared to the 53% of the First World War. An important element of this was due to the reduction in the time it took for the wounded to reach an adequately equipped surgical unit.[3]

References:

1. Owen William Richards in *Plarr's Lives of the Fellows,* The Royal College of Surgeons of England. Online.
2. Combat Casualty Care and Surgical Progress. Ann.
3. Surg. 2006 Jun: 243(6): 715–719.
4. Abdominal surgery in war – the early story. Journal of the Royal Society of Medicine. Volume 84 September 1991.

1915. USA. Intracranial surgery for missile injuries in wartime.

In 1915, three American Universities, Harvard, Western Reserve University and Pennsylvania sent surgeons to set up a military hospital in France. This was organised by Professor Harvey Cushing (1869–1939), a famous American surgeon. He returned in 1917 with the American Army after the USA had declared war on Germany. It was in France that Cushing pioneered operations to remove missile fragments lodged in the brain. He recorded that in one 24-hour period the hospital dealt with 499 casualties. He kept detailed records and operated upon thousands of men to remove intracranial foreign bodies. To aid this endeavour, he developed a powerful magnet to retrieve metallic fragments from the brain where possible.[1]

This was not a new idea, for in 1830 Dr William Gunn(1804–1890) RN, a medical officer in the British Royal Navy ordered a magnet to remove iron filings from the workers eyes at the great shipbuilding port of Chatham. This was the time when the Royal Navy began to build warships of iron rather than timber.[2]

References:

1. Combat Casualty Care and Surgical Progress. Ann. Surg. 2006 Jun: 243(6): 715–719.

2. His was not a surgical case, it was not my duty to attend to him: The Surgeons Role in 19th century Dockyards by Richard Biddle. Pub Med Central Canada. Med History 2013, Oct. 58 (4), 559–588.

1918. England. Total Cystectomy.

The first total excision of the urinary bladder (cystectomy) was in 1918 and is attributed to Mr John C Jefferson (1888–1954) a surgeon at Rochdale Infirmary[1] in England. In 1949, Mr Terrence John Millin (1903–1980) a consultant Urologist at the Royal Masonic Hospital, London carried out a total transabdominal cystectomy with special attention to the anatomical and pathological principles involved.[2 & 3] In 1987, Drs Peter N. Schlegal and P.C Walsh mapped the neuroanatomy of the pelvic plexus enabling surgeons to avoid damaging it where possible to preserve sexual function.[4]

The mortality was initially 5–10% following surgery but has since been reduced to 1–2%. Approximately, 31,000 new cases of bladder cancer were recorded in 1996 in the USA. Egyptian men are at especial risk of developing squamous celled carcinomas caused by Schistoma haematobium infesting the bladder.

Following a total-cystectomy, a urinary conduit is needed and in modern times the commonest method is to implant the ureters into one end of an isolated segment of the ileum, with the other end brought out onto the skin in the right lower quadrant of the abdomen as an ileostomy. Urine is then collected in a bag. The urinary conduit is a part of a group of original operations discussed under reconstructive gut surgery.[5]

References:

1. Total Excision of Urinary Bladder. The Lancet, Vol. 192, No. 4927, P 815–816. 14th Dec1918.
2. Total Cystectomy. A consideration of Technique by Terrance Millin, Wiley Online Library, BJUI. First published June 1949.
3. Terrance John Millin. *Plarr's Lives,* The Royal College of Surgeons of England, online.
4. Schlegal PN, Walsh PC Neuroanatomical approach to radical cysto-prostatectomy with preservation of sexual function. J Urol. 1987 Dec138(6): 1402–6.

5. This Chapter. 1969. Reconstructive gut surgery.

1919. USA. Hiatus hernia repair and surgery for gastro-oesophageal reflux.

Hiatus hernia was first recognised as a pathological entity in the 1850s. An earlier post-mortem review found 88 cases from before 1900 that clearly demonstrated the gastro-oesophageal junction and found that three of these had para-oesophageal hernias. After 1900, X-rays were used to diagnose the condition and the original operation to reduce a hiatus hernia was by Dr Angelo L. Soresi[1] (1877–1951) of New York in 1919.

In 1926, Dr Ackerland described different types of hiatus hernias. There were patients with a congenitally short oesophagus, those with a para oesophageal gastric hernia and other types of hernia. The physiological link between the presence of a hiatus hernia and reflux of acid into the oesophagus was not made until the second half of the 20th century when it was realised that an anatomical repair alone was not sufficient.

Mr Norman Rupert Barrett (1903–1989), a Thoracic surgeon at St Thomas' Hospital, London, focussed on the restoration of the gastro-oesophageal angle to prevent reflux. Hiatus hernia surgery then began to change from an anatomical repair to a physiological restoration of function. It was then recognised that the junction between the oesophagus and stomach acted as a flutter valve to prevent gastric acid refluxing into the oesophagus when abdominal pressure was raised, as in severe exercise or when lying flat. Manometry was later introduced as a useful test to evaluate the results of surgery by comparing the pre- and post-operative readings of acid in the lower oesophagus.[2]

Mr Rudolph Nissen (1896–1981) and Mr Ronald Belsey (1910–2007), both thoracic surgeons in Bristol, England had by 1955 developed what became known as the 'Nissan fundoplication', that was copied by most surgeons in the second half of the 20st century.

These operations are now carried out through a laparoscopic approach. More recently a new prosthesis is being tested by inserting a 'Magnetic Sphincter Augmentation' around the lower oesophagus to achieve the same result.[3] After 40 months, the initial trials were satisfactory. There needs to be a note of caution, as the similar Angelchik[4] prosthesis of the 1980s was ultimately a failure.

References:

1. The History of Hiatal Hernia Surgery. Nicholas Stylopoulos and David W. Ratner. Annals of Surgery. 2005 Jan: 241(1): 185–193.
2. The History of Hiatal Hernia surgery. Nicholas Stylopoulos & David W. Rattnee. Ann Surg. 2005 Jan: 241(1): 185–193.
3. Introduction into the NHS of magnetic sphincter augmentation; an innovative surgical therapy for reflux – results and challenges. D. Prakash, B. Campbell, S. Wajed. Annals RCS of England. Vol 100. Issue 4 April 2018. p 251–256.
4. Complications of the Angelchik prosthesis. NCBI. https://www.ncbi.nlm.nih.gov

1923. USA. Development of angiography.

In 1923, Dr Barney Brooks (1888–1952) in the USA initiated clinical vascular radiography by injecting sodium iodine into a femoral artery to reveal disease in the femoral and popliteal arteries[1] of the leg.

Then in 1927, Dr Antonio Egas Moniz (1874–1955), a neurologist in Lisbon further developed angiography by injecting radio-opaque dyes and then took X-rays of the cerebral arteries. This led to the identification of internal carotid artery occlusion and other arterial lesions. His techniques of arteriography and venography are now used worldwide. He was awarded the Nobel Prize for Physiology or Medicine[2] in 1949.

References:

1. Brooks B. Intra-arterial injection of sodium iodide and study of the femoro-popliteal arteries. JAMA. 1924: 82: 1016–1019.
2. Wikipedia. Antonio Egas Moniz.

1923. USA. Mitral valve repair. First successful open-heart operation.

In 1923, Dr Elliott Cutler (1888–1947) of the Peter Bent Brigham Hospital in the USA reported a successful mitral valve operation in a child with rheumatic mitral valve stenosis. The operation was carried out by dilating the mitral valve with a finger.[1]

Earlier, an operation bordering on open heart surgery was carried out in 1891 by Dr Henry C Dalton of St Louis, USA, who repaired a torn pericardium in a patient who had been stabbed in the chest. A similar operation was carried by Dr Daniel Hale Williams of Chicago two years later.[2 & 3]

By the 1960s, the surgical option of choosing between a mitral valvotomy or mitral valve replacement became possible when the heart-lung machine was introduced in the 1950s. This apparatus revolutionised cardiac surgery as it maintained the circulation of the patient's blood while the heart was stopped and enabled all the subsequent major cardiac surgical operations to be developed.

The traditional approach to gain access to the heart was by splitting the sternum, in the 21st century this approach has been challenged by a minimally invasive thoracoscopic approach. This is not mentioned in 'General Surgery Lecture Notes' published in 2011, as minimally invasive approaches for this operation have not yet proved to be adventageous.[4]

References:

1. Cardiac Surgery. Texas Heart Inst. J. Dr Allen B. Weisse. 2011: 38(5). P. 486–490.
2. Department of Cardiovascular Surgery, Mount Sinai Hospital, 1190 Fifth Avenue, New York, NY. 866-MITRAL5 (648–7255).
3. *The End of the Golden Age of General Surgery: 1870–2000.* By Nigel Keith Maybury. Amazon Independent Publishing Platform. ISBN 1499531370. 2014. p 80–81.
4. *General Surgery Lecture Notes* by Harold Ellis, Sir Roy Calne and Christopher Watson. Wiley Blackwell, 2011.

1925. Austria. Parathyroidectomy.

Dr Felix Mandel (1892–1958) of Vienna was the first surgeon to electively excise a parathyroid adenoma in a patient with advanced osteitis fibrosa cystica (OFC). OFC occurs when pathologically high levels of parathormone causes mobilisation of calcium from the bones. This can result in the formation of lacunae, areas in bones where all the calcium has been completely reabsorbed, that are easily identified by an X-ray. They cause weakness in the bone, frequently resulting in pathological fractures.

In the 1960s, the development of routine biochemical assays of blood samples led to the earlier diagnosis of raised serum calcium levels. This enabled earlier surgery to avoid the development of lacunae and subsequent fractures. Exploration of both sides of the neck is the operation of choice, for in 95% of patients with hyperparathyroidism only one of the four glands is adenomatous.[1, 2 & 3]

Historically, it was only in 1852 that a parathyroid gland, situated in intimate contact with the thyroid was first identified in a rhinoceros by Professor Richard Owen (1804–1892), the Hunterian Professor and Conservator of the Museum of the Royal College of Surgeons of England. The function of the parathyroid glands was not established until the twentieth century.[4]

References:

1. Surgical treatment of primary Hyperparathyroidism. Indian J Surg. 2014 Aug: 308–315.
2. *Bailey and Love's Short Practice of Surgery* by A.J. Harding-Rains & H. David Richie. H.K. Lewis and Co. Ltd. 1987.
3. *The End of the Golden Age of General Surgery: 1870–2000.* By Nigel Keith Maybury. Amazon Independent Publishing Platform. ISBN 1499531370. 2014. p 47, 173.
4. Richard Owen and the discovery of the parathyroid glands. By Cave A.G.E. Editor Underwood, E.A. *Science, Medicine and History, essays of the evolution of scientific thought and medical practice, written in honour of Charles Singer.* Vol. 2. 1953. London. Oxford University Press. p 217–222.

1929. England. Discovery of penicillin.

In 1929, penicillin was discovered by Sir Alexander Fleming (1881–1955), Professor of Pathology at St Mary's Hospital, London. He also recognised its antimicrobial properties and was awarded a Nobel Prize[1] in 1945 for his discovery.

Professor Howard Walter Florey (1898–1968), Professor of Pathology at Oxford University and Dr Ernst Chain (1906–1989), also a biochemist at Oxford, followed up Fleming's discovery. By 1940, they had produced enough penicillin to prevent infection in mice given an otherwise lethal dose of Staphylococcus aureus.

In December 1941, the USA joined the Allies at war with Germany. It was then that American pharmaceutical companies undertook the industrial manufacture of penicillin. Penicillin as a topical treatment had been available during the Allied invasion of Sicily in 1943. When the allied armies of the USA, Britain and Canada landed on the beaches of Normandy in 1944, they took with them a million doses of injectable penicillin to treat the wounded. This was the first industrial production of an antibiotic. Sir Howard Florey was awarded a Nobel Prize in 1945.[2]

Before the manufacture of penicillin, a red azo aniline dye called Prontosil, of low toxicity and commonly known as a sulphonamide had been produced in 1935. It was discovered by Dr Gerhardt Domagk (1895–1964) and it was active against Group A β-Haemolytic Streptococcus pyogenes infections, which when untreated carry a high mortality. Prontosil was used during the Spanish Civil War and World War Two. In 1939, Gerhardt Domagk was awarded a Nobel Prize in Medicine. Prontosil was discovered by testing thousands of compounds related to azo dyes.[3] In 1937, May and Baker, known as M & B, launched sulfapyridine, another sulphonamide antibacterial. These drugs were finally eclipsed by the wide spectrum activity of penicillin and other antibiotics but remained on the market until the 1960s. Perhaps sulphonamides and bacteriophages will be reassessed in the evolutionary war with antibiotic resistant pathogenic organisms.[4]

The first record of bacterial resistance to penicillin was in 1967, only 24 years after it had become widely available. Pathogenic bacteria can evolve resistant strains faster than new antibiotics can be discovered. The European Centre for Disease Prevention and Control have calculated that in 2015, there were over 671,000 serious antibiotic resistant infections in the European Union and the EU Economic Area.[5] These infections resulted in 33,110 deaths, most of which took place in hospitals. In 2020, antibiotic resistance was continuing to increase without any solution to this problem being found.

Sepsis remains a growing threat to surgery and it is a sobering thought to consider that less than a century ago, even a finger infection, caused by Streptococcus pyogenes, could spread and cause death from septicaemia, which brings to mind the millions who died of sepsis before the discovery of antibiotics.[6]

References:

1. Wikipedia. Sir Alexander Flemming.
2. Wikipedia. Sir Howard Florey.
3. Wikipedia. Discovery of prontosil.
4. Are Viruses the Best weapon for Fighting Superbugs. March 6, 2019. Source Nature Briefing. The Conversation, Academic Rigour, journalistic flair.
5. Wikipedia; Antibiotic resistance.
6. *The End of the Golden Age of General Surgery. 1870–2000. The training and practice of a general surgeon in the late twentieth century*. By N.K. Maybury. Published by Amazon Independent Publishing Platform. 2014, p 101–102 and 175–177.

1929. Germany. Vascular catheterisation leading to endovascular arterial stenting.

Open arterial surgery began to be replaced by endovascular angioplasties and later stenting of arteries. The first human cardiac catheterisation was carried out by Dr Werner Forssmann (1904–1989) of Eberswald in Germany in 1929. He carried out experiments on himself and showed that the right atrium and ventricle could be visualised radiographically following injection of an iodine solution via a catheter inserted into one of his cephalic veins.[1]

By 1941, catheter techniques were also being used to measure cardiac output. In 1956, Dr Werner Forssmann shared a Nobel Prize with Drs Andre Frederic Cournand (1895–1980) and Dickinson W. Richards (1895–1973).

Cournand stated in his acceptance speech that, cardiac catheterisation had been the key in the lock of this discovery.[2] A worldwide registry was set up to record all trans-luminal-coronary angioplasties from 1987.

Coronary arteries with severe atheroma carry a high risk of a heart attack or death. From 1986, it was possible to have a metal stent inserted to reopen an artery and restore coronary artery perfusion. This technique was invented by Dr Jacques Puel (1949–2008) of Toulouse in France and by 2001, almost two million angioplasties had been performed worldwide, with an estimated annual increase of 8%.[3]

Meanwhile in 1990, the first abdominal aortic aneurysm stent graft was carried out by Dr Juan C. Parodi (1942–) in Buenos Aires, Argentina.[4] By 2010, stenting of aortic aneurysms accounted for 78% of all non-ruptured aortic aneurysm interventions worldwide.

References:

1. Werner Forssmann and catheterisation of the heart. Ann Thorac Surg. 1990 Mar: 49(3): 498–9.
2. Hollmann, Wildor (2006). Werner Forssmann, Eberswalde, the 1956 Nobel Prize for Medicine. Eur. J. Med. Res. 11 (10): 409–12.
3. Serruys PW, Kutryk MJB, Ong ATL. Coronary-artery stents. *N Engl J Med* 2006; 354:483–95.
4. 1992: Parodi, Montefiore, and the first abdominal aortic aneurysm stent graft in the United States. Ann Vasc. Surg. 2005 Sept: 19(5): 749–51.

1935. USA. The discovery of heparin.

The major complications that cause postoperative morbidity and mortality are sepsis,[1] dehydration,[2] haemorrhage[3] and pulmonary embolism following deep vein thrombosis. Heparin was first discovered by Dr Jay McLean (1890–1958) and Dr William Henry Howell (1860–1945) in 1916 at Johns Hopkins Hospital in Baltimore in the USA. It was originally isolated from canine liver cells, hence its name. The first clinical trials in the 1930s established heparin to be a safe and effective anticoagulant and was used initially to treat patients with deep vein thrombosis (DVT), pulmonary embolism, unstable angina and acute peripheral arterial occlusions.[4]

In the late 1980s, unfractionated heparin was given subcutaneously to patients as prophylaxis to prevent DVT and pulmonary embolism following surgery. In 1986, low molecular weight heparin largely replaced unfractionated heparin, as it produces a more predictable anticoagulant response. On account of this, it is now used routinely to prevent DVTs.

In 2001, a trial of low molecular weight heparin administered pre and post operatively showed that although 9.4% of 468 patients undergoing colorectal surgery developed a degree of deep vein thrombosis following an operation, only one suffered a non-fatal pulmonary embolism.[3] Since then, the use of prophylactic heparin has prevented innumerable deaths from massive post-operative pulmonary embolism, that in earlier times caused the death of many patients including young adults.[5]

References:

1. Chapter 2. Sepsis. 1865 and 1929.
2. Chapter 2. Dehydration. 1902.
3. Chapter 2. Haemorrhage. 1915.
4. Wikipedia. Discovery of heparin.
5. Subcutaneous Heparin Versus Low Molecular Weight Heparin as Thromboprophylaxis in Patients Undergoing Colorectal surgery. Ann Surg. 2001 Mar: 233(3): 438–444.

1940. USA. The Visualisation of internal organs by ultrasound.

In 1940, Professor Floyd Firestone (1898–1986), Professor of Acoustic Physics at the University of Michigan, built a 'Supersonic Reflectoscope'. This first ultrasonic echo-imaging device was used to detect flaws in metal castings. Later Drs Karl Theo Dussik (1908–1968) and his brother, Freidreich, in 1942 used ultrasound technology to image the human brain. In the 1980s, one of the highest clinical demands for ultrasonic imaging was to identify gallstones. Since then, technology has steadily improved and ultrasound is now widely used in obstetrics, vascular surgery and for diagnosis of intra-abdominal and thoracic disease.

Ultrasound utilises sound waves beyond the range of human hearing at 20,000 Hz or above. The echoes of ultrasound pulses are reflected from different tissues at different frequencies and these are displayed in real time as images. Different sonographic instruments can display two and three-dimensional images and also measure blood flow and the stiffness of tissues.[1]

Reference:

1. Wikipedia. Medical ultrasound.

1943. USA. Vagotomy for chronic duodenal ulcer disease.

In 1910, I.P. Pavlov (1849-1936), the famous Russian physiologist, was the first to prove that the vagal nerves carry both motor and secretomotor impulses to the stomach. He discovered that dividing these nerves in a dog stopped acid secretion in the stomach.[1] In this way Pavlov, unknown to himself, had carried out useful animal trials before the operation to reduce gastric acid secretion in humans was undertaken over thirty years later.

The first recorded truncal vagotomy in humans was carried out by Dr A. Exner, in France in 1912 for a completely different purpose. This was an attempt to alleviate the severe abdominal pain caused during a 'tabetic crisis'. This occurs in patients suffering from quaternary syphilis, a common condition at that time. Syphilis causes demyelination of both the sympathetic and parasympathetic nervous systems.[2]

In 1943, Dr Lester Reynold Dragstedt (1893–1975) and Dr F.M. Owens in the USA divided the vagal nerves to the stomach through a thoracic incision. They were treating patients suffering from chronic duodenal ulcer disease. The vagal nerves innervate the parietal or acid secreting cells of the stomach, so when these nerves are divided, the secretion of gastric acid ceases. It is not an easy operation, as every nerve-fibre, of which there can be many, must be divided for the operation to be successful in preventing secretion of gastric acid. Because of this, only patients who had had suffered with a chronic duodenal ulcer for many years were offered surgery. It was said at that time that patients had to 'earn their vagotomy'.

Following longstanding inflammation, some patients developed significant scarring of the duodenum due to their ulcer. As scar tissue matures, it contracts and becomes stiffer and so narrows the duodenum. The vagal nerves also carry nerve fibres to the muscles of the stomach. The combination of chronic scarring, along with paralysis of the stomach muscles following division of the vagal nerves, resulted in the stomach being unable to empty properly following the operation. The resulting residue of liquid caused persistent vomiting in a stomach unable to empty. To avoid this, an abdominal incision was used, as this enabled the vagal nerves to be divided as they pass from the oesophagus to the stomach and at the same operation, a pyloroplasty was carried out. This is a widening of the exit of the stomach into the duodenum to ensure emptying of the stomach's contents.[3]

Duodenal ulcer was a disease of the 20th century. In 1983, it was so common that 1.8 million working days were lost due to the ill health it caused in the UK. The ulcers always healed when the division of the vagal nerves was complete. However, the operation as mentioned was difficult, and if the vagal nerves were not completely divided, the ulcer recurred. The pyloroplasty, the drainage procedure, could result in the patient suffering from 'dumping syndrome'.[4] This occurs because the stomach could now empty a meal very quickly into the small bowel, and if the contents had a high osmolarity, then fluid was sucked from the circulating blood into the gut. This was so rapid that it caused faintness and severe diarrhoea within minutes. These patients then had to undergo further surgery to reverse the pyloroplasty.

In 1982, Helicobacter pylori, a gram-negative bacterium, was found in the stomach and especially in duodenal ulcers. Helicobacter pylori was then identified as the cause of peptic ulcers by Dr Barry J. Marshall (1951–) and Dr Robin Warren (1937–) in Australia. Treating these bacteria with antibiotics together with proton-pump inhibitors to supress acid secretion enables duodenal ulcers to heal. Within ten years of this discovery, the previously common operation of vagotomy for chronic peptic ulceration had been abandoned. This is another example of medical treatment rendering an operation obsolete. Marshall and Warren were awarded the Nobel Prize for Medicine in 2005.[5]

References:

1. *The Works of the Digestive Glands.* Lectures by I.P. Pavlov. Translated by W.H. Thompson. London. Charles Griffin & Company Ltd., Exeter Street, Strand, London, 1910. Lecture 13.
2. Doctoral Thesis, Oxford University. *Vagotomy: Assessment of Adequacy*, by N.K Maybury. Department of Surgical Studies, Middlesex Hospital and Medical School, London, 1980.
3. *The End of the Golden Age of General Surgery. 1870–2000. The training and Practice of a General Surgeon in the Late Twentieth Century* by N.K. Maybury. Published by Amazon, 2014, p. 120.
4. Dumping syndrome in After Vagotomy, by William and Cox.
5. Barry Marshall. Wikipedia.

1943. USA. Fallot's tetralogy, correction of a congenital cardiac anomaly.

Professor Alfred Blalock (1899–1964) Professor of Surgery at Johns Hopkins University in Baltimore in the USA, assisted by Mr Vivien Theodore Thomas (1910–1985) his surgical technician, used dogs to develop the operative procedures used to treat 'blue baby syndrome'. The operation has become known as the Blalock-Thomas-Taussig shunt operation, it was designed to bypass the pulmonary artery stenosis element of the congenital anomaly of the heart known as Fallot's tetralogy.[1]

The operation had been suggested by Dr Helen Brook Taussig (1898–1986) an American paediatric cardiologist. The research programme lasted for two years. The first surgical correction of Fallot's tetralogy was in 1943, when Blalock considerably assisted by Thomas operated on a fifteen-month-old baby with this congenital anomaly. A right-subclavian artery to pulmonary artery shunt was carried out that enabled the baby's arterial blood to be oxygenated. Vivian Thomas was later awarded an Emeritus Doctorate in recognition of his considerable contribution to this operation and was the first Afro-American to be so recognised.

A year later in 1944, Blalock with Dr Edward A. Park (1877–1969), Professor of Paediatrics at Johns Hopkins Hospital developed a bypass operation for coarctation of the aorta.[2] In 1947, this operation was also carried out at Guy's Hospital in London. By 1948, Blalock created a technique for overcoming another congenital defect, the transposition of the great blood vessels of the heart. In the twenty-first century, coarctation of the aorta may become treatable by balloon angioplasty or open excision with end-to-end anastomosis or by the insertion of an aortic graft.[3] These later operations, brilliant as they are, have not been designated as original operations. Because once Blalock and Thomas had successfully corrected one cardiac anomaly, the correction of others followed this lead.

References:

1. *Bailey & Love's Short Practice of Surgery.* Revised by A.J. Harding Rains and H. David Richie. H.K. Lewis and Co. 1977. Page 747.
2. Wikipedia. Alfred Blalock and Edwards S. Parks.
3. *General Surgery Lecture Notes* by Harold Ellis, Sir Roy Calne and Christopher Watson. Publisher Wiley-Blackwell, 2011.

1943. USA. The dawn of Nuclear Medicine.

Dr Sam M. Seidlin (1895–1955), at Montefiore Hospital in New York, was the first to successfully treat metastases with radioactive iodine in a patient who had previously undergone a thyroidectomy for cancer. Low doses of radioactive iodine are also used to form an image of the thyroid gland to measure its function[1].

Reference:

1. The beginning of radioiodine therapy for metastatic thyroid carcinoma: a memoir of Samuel M. Seidlin. Cancer Biother Radiopharm. 1999 Apr: 14(2): 71–79.

1948. France. First arterial bypass graft.

In 1948, Dr J. Kunlin[1] a French surgeon successfully operated on a patient with a necrotic ulcer of the foot due to an atheromatous occlusion of the femoral artery. He carried out a femoro-popliteal bypass graft, using the patient's own saphenous vein for the bypass. After harvesting it, the vein was reversed to prevent the one-way venous valves stopping the flow of arterial blood. This was an original operation.

This was followed by the first coronary artery bypass graft carried out on the 2nd May 1960 by Dr Robert H. Goetz[2] (1910–2000) and Dr Michael Roman in the USA. Coronary bypass grafting has not been designated as an original operation, because the previous operation by Dr Kunlin had demonstrated that bypass surgery of blocked arteries was possible and had already been carried out successfully.

The Vietnam War of 1954–1983 saw rapid advances in vascular surgery. An analysis of 304 wounded soldiers with major arterial injuries, recorded that 269 were repaired. Vein or homologous arterial grafts were used in 82 cases. Initially, 20% came to amputation, by the end of the war the amputation rate had fallen to 8%. It was also when reliable synthetic grafts made from Dacron (PET) became available. These techniques were developed by Dr Michael Ellis Debakey (1908–2008) of the Department of Surgery, Baylor University College of Medicine, USA. Debakey was probably the most famous vascular surgeon of the 20th century; his success in this area of expertise was forged in the crucible of war, for the new specialty of peripheral vascular surgery was pioneered by him and others in the conflicts of the second half of the 20th century.[3]

Going back to the First World War (1914–1918), damaged and bleeding blood vessels were surgically treated with ligation. If the bleeding artery was a major limb artery, then almost inevitably an amputation followed. In this respect, at that time, treatment had not advanced from that of Celsus (c25 AD) 1900 years before.[4]

When in the latter part of World War II (1939–1945) Dr Debakey and Dr F. A. Simeone analysed 2,471 cases of vascular limb injuries, they recorded that 50% were amputated, while repair of the artery was only attempted in 3% of cases.[5]

This takes us full circle back to the Korean War when the US army medical policy was still to ligate bleeding arteries if a simple end-to-end anastomosis was not possible. Before April 1952, ligation of major arteries was still routine and amputations common. It was at this time that helicopters were first used to bring the wounded rapidly to Mobile Army Surgical Hospitals (MASH) which Debakey had designed. This led to the wounded being operated on more quickly, vital for those whose wounds had cut off the blood supply to a limb.[6]

References:

1. Historical Vignettes in Vascular Surgery. The History of in situ saphenous vein bypass. By John E. Connolly. Editor Norman M Rich. J Vasc Surg, 2011; 53: 241–4.
2. Wikipedia. Dr Robert H. Goetz.
3. Combat Casualty Care and Surgical Progress. Ann. Surg. 2006 Jun: 243(6): 715–719.
4. Chapter 2. c30 AD, Celsus.
5. DeBakey, M. D. and F. A. Simeone: Battle Injuries of Arteries in World War 11. Ann. Surg., 123:534, 1946
6. Annals of Vascular Surgery. Michael S. Baker. May 2016, Vol.33:258–262, doi: 1016/j.avsg.2016.01.010.

1950. England. Eye surgery, the first implant of a synthetic intraocular lens.

Sir Nicholas Harold Ridley[1] (1906–2001) was a Consultant Eye Surgeon at St Thomas's Hospital and Moorfields Eye Hospital in London. During World War II, he saw a wounded fighter pilot with an eye injury, caused when a piece of Perspex from his aircraft's windscreen, shattered by enemy fire had lodged in one eye. Ridley noted that his patient's sight was quite good due to the lucidly of the foreign body and also that there was no evidence of infection. This gave Ridley the idea of replacing a cataract with a Perspex prosthesis. After a great deal of experimental work, he implanted the first synthetic lens into a patient's eye in 1950. His discovery was a life changing original operation that has subsequently seen eyesight restored to millions of patients.

In 1986, Dr Patricia Bath[2] (1942–) invented the Laserphaco Probe, a medical device that improves on the use of lasers to remove cataracts. The first foldable lens implant was devised in 1988 by Ka-yr-Zhou.

Ridley was an example of the discouragement and objections received by a surgeon whose contemporaries did not believe in what he was trying to do. As already mentioned, this was not an uncommon reaction to trailblazers of original operations. His work was later publicly recognised when in 1986, he was made a Fellow of the Royal Society and awarded a knighthood.[3]

References:

1. PubMed**.** Biog. Mem. Fellows R Soc2007; 53. 285–307.
2. Wilson, Donald: Jane Wilson (June 20 2003), The Pride of African American History. AuthorHouse. p 25. ISBN 988-1-4107-2873-9.
3. Plarr's Lives of the Fellows. The Royal College of Surgeons of England. Ridley, (Sir) Nicholas Harold Lloyd (1906–2001).

1950. USA. First kidney transplant, also first whole organ transplant.

On 17th June 1950, Dr Richard M. Lawler (1896–1982), surgeon at the Little Company of Mary Hospital in the United States, carried out the first kidney transplant. His patient aged 49 had polycystic kidneys, one was non-functioning and the other had only 10% of normal function. Lawler wrote in the Time Magazine issue of the 3rd of July 1950, 'It was a desperate experiment on a woman doomed to die because both kidneys were hopelessly diseased'.

Lawler carried out experimental transplants on dogs in preparation for this operation. Ruth Tucker's kidney transplant functioned well for five years before failing. This was before tissue typing and anti-tissue rejection treatment. She survived another five years, as the remaining original kidney had improved slightly in the meantime. Curiously, Dr Lawler showed no further interest in kidney transplantation and continued with his normal practice. He was an unsuccessful nominee for a Nobel Prize in 1982.[1&2] Lawler's kidney transplant was the original operation for organ transplants as will be discussed.

In 1954, Dr Joseph Edward Murray(1919–2012), at the Peter Bent Brigham Hospital in Boston in the USA performed a transplant between identical twins, so avoiding the risk of rejection.[3] Tissue typing was introduced by 1962 accompanied by cyclosporine as an early immunosuppressant. By 1984, about 10,000 kidney transplants had taken place using drugs such as Imuran to suppress rejection. In 2011, 2500 kidneys were transplanted in the United Kingdom. However, twice that number of patients were on dialysis awaiting transplant. The one-year survival of kidney transplant patients was 90–95% and the five-year survival 70–80%.[4]

Other historical footnotes include a successful transplant of a kidneys in a dog in Vienna in 1902. The first human to human transplant that immediately failed due to rejection was in 1933. In 1940, Sir Peter Medawar (1915–1987) at the University of London discovered the immunological basis for tissue rejection and in 1958, Dr Jean Dausset (1916–2009) a French physician described the first leucocyte antigen which enabled sophisticated tissue matching.[5]

The kidney was the first whole organ transplant and is therefore the generic original operation for all subsequent whole or in the case of the gut, partial organ transplants. All these subsequent transplants require great skill to carry them out, but all follow the same pattern of surgery as for kidney transplants. They all require reconnection of the arterial input and venous output to the transplant organ, followed by the other necessary connections. In the case of the kidney, the implantation of the ureter into the bladder and for the liver the reconnection of the portal vein and bile duct. That kidney transplantation was possible gave encouragement to surgeons that other organ transplants could also be successful.

References:

1. *Organ Transplantation* by David Petechuck, Greenwood Publishing Group, USA, 2006. p 11.
2. Kidney Transplant. Little Company of Mary Hospital (online) 1950.
3. Wikipedia. Joseph Edward Murray.
4. *General Surgery Lecture Notes* by Harold Ellis, Sir Roy Calne and Christopher Watson. Wiley-Blackwell 2011.

5. History web.stanford.edu. Kidney Transplantation past, present and future.

1953. USA. Bariatric surgery.

Morbid obesity became a problem in the USA during the first half of the 20th century and in Europe after the Second World War, when food rationing was no longer necessary. It has now developed into a worldwide epidemic.

The first operation to reduce obesity was in 1953 when Dr John H. Linner (1918–2013) a Surgeon in Iowa, USA, carried out an operation to effectively defunction a large portion of the small bowel, with the aim of significantly reducing the amount of food absorbed from the gut. This operation proved successful and was still being practiced in the 1980s, unfortunately it tended to cause metabolic complications in a number of patients.[1&2]

Many different operations were tried after this, including a staple-banded gastroplasty. This was to create a very small pouch from the upper portion of the stomach where it joins the oesophagus, so creating a mini stomach within the stomach. The idea was that patients would eat less as the small pouch would distend and the sensation of fullness would discourage further eating.[3] This operation has not survived the test of time and is now obsolete.

Morbid obesity has continued to increase in the West to such an extent that dedicated Bariatric Surgical Centres are now commonplace. Between 2009 and 2010, the National Bariatric Surgical Registry in the United Kingdom audited the results of 8710 patients who had undergone bariatric surgery. The survey involved 86 hospitals and revealed that two thirds of the patients had a preoperative body mass index (BMI) of more than 50. In the 12 months following the operation, patients lost 60% of their excess weight and 85% of those with pre-operative diabetes were cured. The operations used were gastric bypass surgery, gastric band and sleeve gastrectomy. The results confirmed that bariatric operations were satisfactory both by an open operation and the laparoscopic approach. The laparoscopic technique became the normal surgical approach to treatment in the 21st century.[4]

More recently, non-surgical techniques for mechanically reducing weight loss have been used. Several of them involved a soft balloon or a bag being inserted into the stomach that was then filled with saline. This reduces the capacity of the stomach to accommodate much food and can stay in place for up to four months before being replaced. In 2017, the Food and Drugs

Administration in the USA warned of 12 deaths related to these devices of which the most common was perforation of the stomach occurring within a few weeks of being inserted. Nearly 300,000 of these devices have been used worldwide and the mortality is less than 0.01%.[5] The mortality following surgical procedures for morbid obesity is 0.25%.[6] It looks probable that as non-surgical techniques improve the need for surgery will decline.

References:

1. A brief history of bariatric surgery. Gill R. Faria. Porto Biomedical Journal. Volume 2, Issue 3, May-June 2017, Pages 90–92.
2. *The End of the Golden Age of General Surgery, 1870–2000* in Appendix 3, by N.K. Maybury. Published by Amazon 2014, ISBN 1499531370. P. 178–183.
3. Early results of a Canadian laparoscopic sleeve gastrectomy experience, by Carola Behrens, Bao Q. Tang, Brady J. Amson. Can. J. Surg.2011 Apr; 54(2): 138–142.
4. The Royal College of Surgeons of England. First United Kingdom bariatric surgery audit published for 2009 to 2010.
5. https://www.webmd.com June 6th 2018. FDA issues warning.
6. Morbidity after Bariatric Surgery. Mario Morina *et al.,* Annals of Surgery. Volume 246, Number 6, Dec2007.

c1955. England or the USA. The surgery of myelomeningocele (MMC).

It has not been possible to identify an individual surgeon who undertook the original operation for an infant with myelomeningocele, MMC. This was because surgery is only one aspect of a difficult undertaking. Before the introduction of antibiotics in the late 1940s, virtually all infants with spina bifida died of meningitis and even by the end of the 1950s, the survival rate was only 10%. MMC is where a baby's lower spinal cord remains exposed at birth.

Another major problem following closure of the MMC was that excess cerebral-spinal-fluid, CSF, causes the ventricles within the brain to enlarge causing hydrocephalus. In 1952, a one-way shunt was developed to prevent this. The upper end was placed into one of the cerebral ventricles, the tube was then tunnelled under the skin and the lower end was inserted into the peritoneal cavity to drain the excess CSF. A less used alternative was for the lower end to be inserted into a jugular vein. These techniques were successful in controlling the hydrocephalus.[1]

In 1967 at Sheffield University in England, 500 cases of hydrocephalus who had been operated on during the previous seven years were analysed. The conclusion was that all babies with spina bifida, who did not have deformities incompatible with life, should be operated upon between 12 and 48 hours of being born.[2]

Following the development of hydrocephalus, shunts frequently blocked and required revision, also these infants often underwent many orthopaedic operations. Bladder function was often severely impaired due to infection and led to renal failure, the commonest cause of death in the 1980s.

A lengthy debate concerning the ethics of what could be, and what should be done for these infants followed. From this discussion developed the new concept of Bioethics. Gradually, the outcomes of surgical treatment improved.[3] Better shunt design reduced the need for frequent change and 'clean catheterisation' virtually stopped the incidence of bladder infection that had caused renal failure.

Research into the effects on the exposed spinal cord of a foetus in utero with a myelomeningocele, confirmed that the spinal cord showed progressive deterioration over time while in the womb. To try to avoid this the first in-utero foetal operation was performed. It aimed at closing the spina bifida before the baby was born. The results were encouraging, for babies who underwent this operation were less likely to need a shunt after they were born. They also had less severe problems with their legs.[4] This is described under intra-foetal surgery in the entry for 1981.

Myelomeningocele (MMC) was the first anomaly identified in a baby while in its mother's womb to be treated by in-utero surgery.[5]

References:

1. *The End of the Golden Age of General Surgery.* By N.K. Maybury. Amazon Publishing Platform, 2014. p 30.
2. Living with spina bifida: An historical perspective. By Lisa J. Pruitt. Paediatrics. 2012 Aug. 130(2): 181–183.
3. Keller, B.A, and Farmer, D.L. Fetal Surgery for myelomeningocele: history, research, clinical trials and future directions. Minerva paediatr., 2015 Aug: 67(4): 341–356.

4. Hirose, S. and Farmer, D.L. Fetal Surgery for myelomeningocele. 2009 Jun; 36(2): 431–8.
5. Danzer, E. and Adzick, N.S. Fetal surgery for myelomeningocele: patient selection, perioperative management and outcomes. Fetal Diagn Ther. 2011; 30(3): 163–73. And. Chapter 2. 1981.

1958. USA. Introduction of flexible fibre optic endoscopy.

In February 1958, Dr Basil Hirschowitz (1925–2013), of the University of Michigan, USA, passed the first prototype of a fibre-optic endoscope down his own throat. A few days later, he carried out a clinical examination of a patient's oesophagus. In 1954, he began to use fibre-optics and developed a flexible endoscope. This consisted of a bundle of very fine and flexible fibreglass strands that enabled light to be transmitted while maintaining a coherent image when the scope was flexed.

Introduced through the mouth, this flexible endoscope could reach into the naso-pharynx, oesophagus, stomach and duodenum. A similar instrument inserted through the anus could visualise the rectum and whole colon. By 1960, the first production model was available and further refinements over the next two decades made it possible to take photographs through the endoscope. Eventually, extra channels placed within the endoscope enabled biopsies, suction, insufflation of air and squirting of water to take place. It became possible to carry out biopsies and polypectomies in the colon, its usefulness in gastroenterology was immediately established.[1 & 2]

Before endoscopy, open surgery was essential for diagnosing and treating patients with obstructive jaundice. If the jaundice was caused by gallstones blocking the common bile duct, CBD, then the surgeon would carry out a cholecystectomy, to remove the primary source of gallstones and explore the common bile duct to remove the stones causing the jaundice. If the jaundice was caused by a cancer of the bile duct or more commonly of the head of the pancreas, then a surgical bypass was immediately performed to relieve the jaundice. This was a preliminary operation to allow the jaundice to settle with a view to a further operation to remove the head of the pancreas a few weeks later, if that was feasible.

This approach was replaced by using an endoscope to reach the duodenum. When the papilla, the opening of the common bile duct into the duodenum, had been identified it was dilated endoscopically and gallstones removed by passing a wire basket into the CBD to extract them. If the patient's jaundice is caused by cancer, it is usually possible to pass a tube into the CBD alongside the tumour and leave it in place to drain the bile and so relieve the jaundice. This gives time for investigation and subsequent pancreatic surgery if possible.

Another example of therapeutic endoscopy supplanting an operation was in patients with an inoperable cancer of the oesophagus who had difficulty swallowing. The old operation for this was a mini laparotomy to gain access to the stomach which was then opened. This was so a plastic tube, with a long thin tail below it, could be pushed through the mouth into the stomach by the anaesthetist and then grasped by the surgeon when it reached the stomach. The tube was then pulled into the oesophagus to lie alongside the tumour. The long tail was then cut off leaving the lower end of the tube open. This enabled fluids and a liquidised diet to be taken orally. The stomach and abdomen were then closed. This tube had been invented by Drs Mousseau and Babin in France and was the only palliative treatment available until the late 1980s. It was then supplanted by an endoscopic technique to push a wider stent alongside the tumour in the oesophagus from above and so avoid the abdominal operation altogether.[2]

Historically, the first rigid illuminated endoscope was used to examine the larynx and had been developed in 1894 by Dr John Macintyre (1858–1928) at Glasgow Royal Infirmary. Macintyre also set up the World's first Radiology department; he was helped by Glasgow being one of the first hospitals to have mains electricity.[3]

References:

1. Dittrick Medical History Centre 2017, Caes Western Reserve University, Hirschowitz fibreoptic Endoscope, 1960. (2). Wikipedia History of the Fibrescope.
2. *The End of the Golden Age of General Surgery. 1870–2000* by N.K. Maybury. Pub. CreateSpace on Amazon. ISBN. 1499531370. P. 112–114.
3. Wikipedia. Biography of Dr John Macintyre.

1958. USA. Harrington's rods used to treat idiopathic scoliosis.

Dr Paul Randall Harrington(1911–1980), an orthopaedic surgeon at the Jefferson Davis County Hospital in Kansas, USA, devised what became known as Harrington's Rods. His original operation involved the implantation of metal rods alongside the spine to which they were anchored. They were devised to straighten the spine in cases of scoliosis. Harrington presented his work to the American Academy of Orthopaedic Surgeons in Chicago in 1958 where his idea was initially met with deep scepticism, but later accepted.[1]

In 1911, an unsuccessful attempt was made to control deformities of the spine by Dr Russel A. Hibbs (1869–1932) another American orthopaedic surgeon. Untreated scoliotic spines can result in cosmetically and functionally unacceptable rib humps, waist asymmetries, shoulder imbalance and lead to severe cardio-pulmonary impairment. Hibbs found that these deformities could not be controlled by external means and his unsupported fusions also proved unsatisfactory.

Harrington also operated on many children who had suffered polio in the 1940s and 1950s and subsequently developed scoliosis. He successfully introduced a hook-rod system for concave-distraction and convex-compression of the spine in the late 1950s.

By 1983, Dr Yves Cotrel (1925–2019) and Professor Jean Dubousset in France introduced an improved system where none of the patients needed a post-operative brace or cast. New developments are underway and those interested might read Dr Carol C Hasler's article.[2]

References:

1. American Academy of Orthopaedic Surgeons. Arresting development – Dr Paul Harrington MD. Archived on 24th July 2010. However, his operation gradually gained acceptance.
2. A Brief Overview 0f 100 years of History of Surgical Treatment for Adolescent Idiopathic Scoliosis by Carol C Hasler. J Child Orthop. 2013 Feb; 7(1): 58–62.

1961. England. First successful total hip replacement.

In 1961, Sir John Charnley (1911-–1982), Professor of Orthopaedic Surgery at Wrightington Hospital, near Wigan in England, developed and implanted an artificial hip. It consisted of a low friction arthroplasty, with a steel femoral head and neck to replace the head of the femur; this is fitted into a synthetic acetabulum of high molecular weight polyethylene. This provides a stable long-term total hip replacement and still remains the leading prosthesis.[1]

Attempts to develop a synthetic hip began in 1891 when Dr Thermistokles Gluck (1853–1942) implanted an ivory ball and socket which quickly failed. Dr Marius Smith Petersen (1866–1953) of Boston, USA, interposed a vitallium cup into the joint that only worked for a short while. Then the Drs Judet in France, used an acrylic head on a metal stem which worked well initially but the metal stems soon fractured.[2]

A forgotten surgeon who replaced hip joints was Mr Philip Wiles (1899–1967), an orthopaedic surgeon at the Middlesex Hospital in London, who designed and inserted total hip replacements in the 1930s. Wiles' records were destroyed during the bombing of London during the Second World War.

However, one of his patients was reputed to have had his arthroplasty still functioning 35 years later. If this could be verified, Wiles would be the first to have successfully carried out a total hip replacement.[3] His obituary published by the Royal College of Surgeons of England in *Plarr's Lives of the Fellows*, does not mention his work on hip replacements.[4] Also, Mr Austin Moore in 1940 developed a hemi-replacement arthroplasty[5] which was short lived.

Once the principle of successful hip joint replacement had been established by Charnley, other joints began to be replaced. Only Charnley's hip replacement has been designated as an original operation, because the principle of successful joint replacement was established by Charnley. Other joint replacements followed and these are here defined as successor operations, for their authors knew that with perseverance they too could be successful.

Total knee replacement or knee arthroplasty was first carried out in 1968 and accounted for 4.6% of all operations in the USA by 2011.

The first shoulder joint replacement was attempted in 1892 when Dr Jules-Emile Paen (1830–1898), a French surgeon, tried to use a prosthesis to replace a tubercular joint.[6] The modern era of shoulder replacement began with Dr Charles S. Neer II (1917–2011), in the USA who in 1982 designed a humeral component to conform to a polyethylene glenoid prosthesis.[7]

Ankle joint replacements have been undergoing trials in the early 21st century with early success.[8]

References:

1. Charnley J. (1961) Lancet, 1. 1129 (Arthroplasty of the hip, a new operation.
2. Judet J. and Judet R. (1950) J. Bone Jt. Surg., 32B, 166 (The use of an artificial femoral head for arthroplasty of the hip joint).
3. Wikipedia. Philip Wiles.
4. Philip Wiles in *Plarrs Lives* online. The Royal College of Surgeons of England.
5. Moore, A.T. (1952) Sth. med J. (Bgham, Ala), 45, 1015 (Metal hip joint: a new self-locking vitallium prosthesis).
6. History of Hip Resurfacing: the early years. Total Hip Replacement. Online coloradohipresurfacing.com.
7. Wikipedia. Biography of Jules-Emile Paen.
8. Orthopaedics Today on Line. A century of shoulder arthroplasty innovations and discoveries.

1969. England. Reconstructive gut surgery.

1. Anal sphincter reconstruction.

In 1969, Mr Aubrey York-Mason (1910–1993) a surgeon at St Helier's Hospital, London, devised an operation to repair a fistula.[1] In this case, a false passage between the prostatic capsule and rectum. This was an occasional complication following prostatectomy through a suprapubic approach. The fistula resulted in urine leaking from the bladder into the rectum.

The purpose of Mason's operation was to close the fistula. To accomplished this, access to the site where the fistula was situated and leaking urine was necessary. This required access to the front of the rectum just above the anus, so as to be able to operate and close the fistula. To achieve this, it was necessary to completely divide the anal sphincter. Once the fistula was closed, it was then essential to reconstruct the divided anal sphincter with great care to avoid any possibility of subsequent faecal incontinence, which would be disastrous for the patient.

Successful reconstruction of the anal sphincter was dependent on the surgeon identifying each of the sphincter muscles in turn before dividing them. To do this, it was necessary to tie each sphincter muscle in turn with two sutures. Each pair of sutures needed to be of a different colour or type. So, when each sphincter muscle had been divided by cutting between each pair of sutures, both ends of it could still be individually identified. This ensured that when reconstruction of the anal sphincter took place, each muscle was identified by its matching sutures and when tied together, restored them to their correct anatomical position, this re-established normal function. This was an original operation and its success depended on Mason's careful technique.

It is of passing interest that the successful reconstruction of the 'lowly' anus fell to the surgeon's knife at an earlier date than the first heart transplant.

References:

1. Trans-sphincteric exposure of the rectum. Mason AY. Ann R Coll Surg Engl. 1982: 181: 1178–83.
2. *The End of the Golden Age of General Surgery* by N.K. Maybury. Amazon. 2014. ISBN: 1499531370. p 51.

2. Use of small bowel pouches to replace excised rectum, stomach and bladder.

In the mid-1970s, Sir Alan Parks (1920–1982) of St Mark's Hospital, London, pioneered what was called a 'J' pouch. This was fashioned from the terminal ileum to form a reservoir to replace the rectum after it had been excised due to severe ulcerative colitis.[1] The pouch was made from the terminal 30 cm of the ileum, which was then anastomosed to the anus. This procedure was offered to patients about to undergo a pan-proctocolectomy (excision of the colon and rectum) for ulcerative colitis, or more rarely hereditary polyposis coli. The alternative to this operation was and is a permanent ileostomy.

In patients who are acutely ill, the operation is carried out in two stages. The first to remove the diseased colon and over-sew and leave the rectum in place, an ileostomy was formed to allow evacuation of the small bowel into a bag. At the second operation, when the patient was in better health, the rectum was excised leaving the anus intact. The ileostomy was then taken down and a 'J' pouch constructed from the end of it. This was then sutured to the anus.[2] Approximately, 25% of patients with ulcerative colitis require colectomy and the ileo-anal-pouch anastomosis (IPAA) has become the operation of choice, but is not suitable for all patients. There are ongoing trials to compare open surgery with a laparoscopic operation. Significant complications, mainly chronic infection, occur in about 15% of patients.[2 & 3]

From the 1980s, patients who had undergone a total gastrectomy for cancer of the stomach had it 'replaced' by a jejunal pouch, to act as a new reservoir for food, that was anastomosed above to the oesophagus. At the lower end, the duodenum was closed and the jejunum divided, the upper end of the jejunum was then anastomosed to the lower end of the new 'gastric pouch' and the lower end of the duodenum was anastomosed to the jejunum lower down. This is a safe procedure with a favourable perception of quality of life by patients.[4]

The third use of a short section of small bowel is used as a conduit for urine following the total excision of the bladder for cancer. A segment of the ileum is isolated and the ureters are implanted into its upper end while the distal end is brought out as an ileostomy to drain the urine into a bag.[5]

References:

1. Proctocolectomy without ileostomy for ulcerative colitis. Parks AG, Nicholls RJ. Br Med J. 1988. 2: 85–8.
2. Ileal pouch surgery for ulcerative colitis. World J Gastroenterol. 2007 Jun28: 13(24): 3288–3300.
3. Techniques of reconstruction after total gastrectomy for cancer. Lehnert T, Buhl K. Br. J Surg. 2004 May: 91(5): 528–39.
4. *The End of the Golden Age of General Surgery.* By N.K. Maybury. Amazon, 2014. p 49.
5. Uretero-ileal conduit. Modifications of the surgical technique. Draper JW *et al.,* Journal of Urology Nov. 1981; 106(5): 664–7.

1981. USA. First in-utero foetal operation.

Foetal surgical techniques using animal models were carried out in 1980 by Dr Michael R. Harrison (1943–) at the University of California, San Francisco. The first successful human open foetal operation was by Harrison on the 26th April 1981. The foetus had a congenital hydronephrosis with a kidney dangerously distended. A catheter was placed in the ureter to enable release of the urine. The actual cause of obstruction was removed surgically after the birth of the baby.[1]

In 1991, the first in-utero cardiac operation was on a congenitally defective aortic valve. Of the first 12 of these operations, only two survived.

In the 1990s, in-utero closure of myelomeningoceles (MMC) were carried out before 26 weeks of gestation. Closing the spinal defect did succeed in preserving and improving neurological function of the legs. The operation also prevented hindbrain herniation and also avoided the need for a cerebro-ventricular peritoneal shunt after the infant was born, as the incidence of hydrocephalus was significantly reduced. These studies unfortunately revealed that foetal surgery is associated with significant maternal and foetal risks. Further research is being undertaken to understand the pathophysiology of MMC.[2&3]

References:

1. Wikipedia. Foetal Surgery. 1981. Hydronephrosis.
2. Danzer, E. and Adzick, N.S. Fetal surgery for myelomeningocele: patient selection, perioperative management and outcomes. Fetal Diagn Ther. 2011; 30(3): 163–73.
3. See this Chapter, c1955.

Chapter 13
Analysis of Surgery in the Fifth Period

1. General anaesthesia.
2. Surgical training in this Period.
3. Impact of science and technology on diagnosis and treatment.
4. The causes of operative morbidity and mortality.
5. Countries where original operations took place.
6. Technical advances that made surgery safer.
7. Whole organ excisions dominated surgery at the start of this period.
8. The increasing complexity of surgery.
9. Further development of original operations in this period.
10. Transplant operations.
11. Summary.

1. General anaesthesia

The availability of general anaesthesia after 1846 enabled every part of the body to undergo pre-planned and unhurried operations. Speed of operating was no longer an indication of surgical skill as it had been in earlier times, as when Mr Robert Liston[1] (1794–1847), an accomplished Scottish surgeon, earned himself the soubriquet of 'The fastest knife in the West', when he amputated a leg in two and a half minutes.

Within weeks of its introduction in the USA, anaesthetics were being given for minor surgery in England and continental Europe.[2] However, it took longer for surgeons to adjust and plan major intra-abdominal original operations and seven years were to elapse before the first, a hysterectomy was carried out.

This surgeon carried out another 14 hysterectomies, of which only three survived infection and death mainly from sepsis.[3] It was Sir Frederick Treves in his *Manual of Operative Surgery* of 1892, who quoted a postoperative mortality of 70% for this operation. This tragic outcome for so many patients was not uncommon in the early years of anaesthesia. It was the introduction and use of Lister's antiseptic spray that reduced mortality to 5%. High rates of post-operative mortality did not pass unnoticed. For example, Professor Theodor Billroth (1829–1894)[4] in Austria was stoned by an angry crowd after one of his early gastrectomy patients died. He was lucky to survive. Before anaesthesia patients with serious disease affecting the brain, chest or abdomen, all died of their disease. Nowadays, it is difficult to grasp the precariousness and often shortness of life not so very long ago.

Surgeons also needed to learn and understand the intricacy of internal anatomy so as to be able to operate safely and unlike the past this knowledge was now available. For dissection of cadavers was being carried out regularly in the teaching hospitals, as it became compulsory for medical students to dissect a cadaver to learn the anatomy of the whole body, as it is the 'foundation science' of surgery.

2. Surgical training in this Period.

In 1880, a new approach to training was introduced by Dr William Halstead[5] (1852–1922) in the USA. He established a surgical residency programme for newly qualified doctors. Not long afterwards, a similar programme was introduced in the United Kingdom, this way of teaching surgery proved durable and lasted 120 years until the end of the 20th century.

Halstead's training programme, as it was practiced in the UK, was as follows. To become a consultant surgeon in the second half of the 20th century took 12 to 14 years. To achieve this, students were required to have university degrees in medicine and surgery or the equivalent. They then spent two to three years as a clerk, still as a student learning the practicalities of their profession in a teaching hospital. After qualifying as a doctor, the following years were served in a progression of appointments of increasing responsibility, while working under the direct supervision of two consultant surgeons in a 'Firm' with trainee surgeons of increasing seniority. The young surgeon started as a house officer, the most junior grade and then worked up through the grades to eventually become a senior registrar. After three to four years in this last post, trainees having passed the required exams were eligible to apply for a permanent posting in a hospital as a fully trained consultant surgeon.

Until the beginning of the 21st century, every consultant when appointed had clinical independence to diagnose and treat his or her patients to the best of their ability. All consultants were of equal status in all disciplines, giving them all the satisfaction of being at the top of their profession. With this came great responsibility for each and every patient entrusted to them. This continuing responsibility applied not only when operating, but also in outpatient clinics and on the wards and at night. This was in keeping with the consultant contract of that time that simply demanded and stated that 'at all times' the named consultant had 'a continuing clinical responsibility for patients in your charge'. In those days, the role of managers and administrators was to provide the best facilities possible for consultants to practise. Although consultants worked within the public National Health Service, they practiced independently of management.

Patients usually returned to see their General Practitioner after an operation to check that all was well; this also acted as a form of professional quality control on the work of the consultant surgeon. GPs had the choice and could refer patients to another consultant if they so wished. This freedom in surgical practice continued into the National Health Service when it was established on the 5th of July 1948 and lasted for just over 50 years. For at the turn of the new millennium, the framework for clinical practice changed dramatically.

There were a number of causes that led to this change. The increase in population and longevity meant that patients over 65 made up more than 18% of the population by 2018. With a longer life comes the medical problems of old age with associated multiple degenerative diseases, requiring much more medical attention than the younger population of the past.

There were also changes in the commonest causes of death. In general, during the 1950s and '60s, death was caused by circulatory and coronary artery disease, often associated with chronic respiratory disease and infections. By the beginning of the 21st century, ischaemic heart disease was still the leading cause of death in men, but in women, it has become dementia and Alzheimer's disease. Longevity also brought other diseases of old age, including cancer and degenerative skeletal disease.

This hugely increased the pressure on hospitals and staff due to the sheer numbers of elderly patients needing treatment for multiple degenerative conditions. This acted as a major stimulus to streamline treatment, by training surgeons to work in a strictly focused range of surgery, aimed at their becoming super-specialists in a limited and defined area of expertise. It was anticipated that this would increase the throughput of patients. Also, of great consequence, the training of surgeons was significantly reduced from 80,000 to 6000 hours.[6]

Specialisation was not entirely new and had been the norm nearly 4,000 years ago in Ancient Egypt. In the UK, specialisation was already gathering pace following the introduction of anaesthesia in 1846. In 1850, the Royal College of Surgeons of England was the sole organisation in England that maintained standards and set examinations to test the competence of candidates to become surgeons. During the next century and a half, surgery split into at least 16 specialties, most with their own Associations and each with their own examinations. It is inevitable that this has weakened them all when it comes to negotiations with government who were responsible for shortening the length of training.

As a result, at the beginning of the 21st century the Consultant Contract was changed to recognise that super-specialisation, within a narrow field of expertise was now the norm. This was when the 'surgical firms' were disbanded, resulting in the abandonment of a system of training that was still working well 120 years after its introduction. It was replaced by more formalised academic training with the loss of the former close contact between consultant and his or her trainees, when previously, they would have worked together for six months in the case of a junior house officer, to two or more years for surgical registrars. Trainees had benefitted from being part of a consultant led Firm, by attending ward rounds, out-patients and operating sessions together, where the whole team knew all the patients for whom they were responsible and looked after them together. Of course, the patients also knew who was looking after them.

The factor that actually precipitated this momentous change was the European Union's 'Working Time Directive',[7] that may not have been specifically aimed at the medical profession. It came into force at the end of the last century and imposed a strict working week of 48 hours. It was aimed to ensure that heavy or monotonous work, such as in the building trade or long-haul lorry driving did not result in fatigue and accidents. For surgeons it profoundly affected their pattern of work and the directive was imposed on all the countries within the European Union including the United Kingdom at that time.

Following this, for the first time, it became necessary for doctors to work in shifts to ensure 24-hour cover in hospitals daily throughout the year. Before the implementation of the 'Working Time Directive', most hospitals had several Firms of surgeons. Each Firm usually had two consultants with their junior staff.

Each firm was on duty continuously for emergencies for 24 hours one day a week, weekends were covered by each of the firms in rotation. Even when on duty for emergencies, routine operating lists and outpatients continued as normal. Surgical emergencies were added to the operating list as necessary so surgeons would often work through the night. Emergencies requiring urgent surgery were treated promptly. All the other days of the week were worked normally.

As mentioned, the result of the EU time directive made working in Firms impossible and thereby the close clinical attachment, regular supervision and continuous teaching by consultants of their junior colleagues was lost. For example, before the directive, a new surgical registrar would initially assist at operations of varying complexity, then would carry out part of an operation under direct supervision. Gradually, as their competence and confidence increased, they would be allowed to carry out a whole operation, such as hernia repair, with the consultant in the neighbouring operating theatre who would come through to assist and teach how to handle unusual and difficult problems that can occur in any operation. The key was direct and indirect supervision by the nearby consultant and when he or she had confidence that their junior would immediately call them when they found something difficult so that it could then be solved together. Using this method, the author found that a good registrar, on his busy firm, could operate at a high standard on minor, intermediate and some straight forward major surgery by the end of nine months. This method of training has now been abandoned.

When the National Health Service was established, the number of surgeons in training increased and the majority, when eligible, were appointed to District General Hospitals as consultant surgeons. Their predecessors who were trained before the Second World War usually referred more complex operations to the surgeons at their local teaching hospital. The post-war trained consultant surgeons had a wider range of operations within their competence, which included more complex operations than their predecessors. On account of this, between 1960 and 2000, District General Hospitals reached a peak in the range of operations they were capable of undertaking, enabling them to offer an almost comprehensive service to their local populations. This was the zenith of practice in District General hospitals. It was not to last.

The reorganisation of services in the drive for super specialisation was also accompanied by a cultural change. Resistance was growing among younger surgeons to the long hours worked while training. In some cases, although rare, it could have involved 120 hours on duty and on call during a week.[8] Since no training system is perfect, surgeons in the past were jokingly thought of as being over experienced and under-trained, while now the opposite is true.

Box 13.1.

The progress of Surgical Training during the seven centuries following the Edict of Tours.

1163. The Edict of Tours and the separation of surgery from medicine.[9]

1252. The foundation of the Company of Barber-Surgeons in Paris followed by London[7] in 1308.[10]

1312. Trainee surgeons apprenticed for seven years[11] to a Barber Surgeon.

1768. The development of teaching hospitals[12] in London.

1844. First examination for the Fellowship of the Royal College of Surgeons of England.[13]

1860. The foundation of the Nightingale School of Nursing[14] at St Thomas' Hospital, London, that enabled a high standard of nursing care to be given to patients.

1880. Professor Theodore Billroth (1829–1894)[15] in Vienna trained a generation of surgeons including Dr William J. Halstead (1852–1922)[16] who established a hospital surgical residency programme for trainee surgeons in the USA. This system was soon afterwards introduced into England and replaced the former apprenticeship.

2000–2001. The implementation of the European Union's Working Time Directive imposed a working week of 48 hours that meant doctors had to work in shifts,[17] so ending the former practice of full time working in firms.

3. Impact of science and technology on diagnosis and treatment.

As time passes, it might be expected that patients will tend to present earlier with fewer signs and symptoms of a disease. At the same time, technology of increasing complexity is progressively playing a key role in diagnosis, as recorded in Box 13.2.

Box 13.2.

A brief timeline of science and technology during the fifth period of surgery

1846. Introduction of anaesthesia.[18]

1858. Microorganisms discovered and germ theory of disease confirmed.[19]

1865. Introduction of Lister's anti-septic surgical technique.[20]

1879. The introduction of electricity.[21]

1895. The discovery of x-rays.[22] First clinical x-rays were carried out within six months.

1896. The discovery of radiation[23] led first to secondary treatment of cancers and is now used in some cases as primary treatment.

1899. Introduction of isotonic intra-venous fluids.[24] It was some decades before this was clinically useful.

1908. The invention of electro-diathermy[25] for cutting tissues and coagulating small vessels made operations easier and reduced blood loss. This instrument is the sophisticated successor to the red-hot cautery of the ancient and medieval surgeons.

1910. Introduction of laparoscopy.[26] It was not until 1987 that the first laparoscopic cholecystectomy was carried out.

1915. First clinical blood transfusion.[27]

1923. Development of angiography[28] led to vascular surgery by identifying areas of obstruction in arteries. In 1929, vascular catheterisation was introduced and later angioplasties,[29] leading to the insertion of intra-arterial stents.

1929. Discovery of penicillin.[30] First clinically available in large quantities was at the Normandy landings of the allies in 1943.

1935. Discovery of Heparin.[31]

1940. Invention of ultrasound,[32] Widespread clinical use from 1990.

1957. Introduction of the flexible endoscope[33] revolutionised gastroenterology in terms of diagnosis in general and in the treatment of gastro-intestinal and biliary disease.

1974. CT Scanners[34] became available.

1987. Magnetic Resonance Imaging,[35] now plays a major role in diagnosis of cranial, thoracic and abdominal disease.

2000. The introduction of robotic assisted surgery[36] commenced and its usefulness has since increased.

The shift in treatment away from some aspects of surgery is inevitable. To give one example, patients presenting with obstructive jaundice are now investigated endoscopically rather than surgically.[37] Box 13.3, gives more examples of operations that were formerly essential, but are now obsolete or are likely to become so in the future.

The trend for operations to become obsolete will almost certainly continue to gather pace. As previously noted, in his inaugural lecture at Leicester

University in 1974, Professor Sir Peter Bell[38] suggested to his audience that within 50 years, 'Diseases that are now the province of the surgeon will have either disappeared or become treated by medical means'. Professor Bell has been proved right. As the world population increases, possibly to reach 10 billion before the end of this century, surgeons working in a focused but limited range of operations may find that their operations have been replaced by medical interventionalist procedures. There are of course possible exceptions to this trend, orthopaedic surgery comes to mind as an ageing population with increasing joint failure will require replacements, but even these conditions might be treated medically in the future.

Box 13.3.

Original operations that are obsolete or may become obsolete due to medical treatment and other technological advances.

1. Thyroidectomy for hyperthyroidism was first carried out in 1890.[39] Following the introduction of radioactive iodine in 1942, an increasing number of patients have opted for this treatment rather than surgery.
2. The first laryngectomy for cancer took place in 1873.[40] Now with early diagnosis, these can often be resected endoscopically or ablated by using trans-oral laser microsurgery.
3. In 1903, portal-hypertension caused by cirrhosis of the liver was controlled by a venous bypass shunt. Eighty years later, surgery has been replaced by drugs and endoscopic control of haemorrhage. A bypass is now achieved by an interventionalist medical technique to insert a shunt introduced via the jugular vein.[37] A liver transplant is still the only operation for end stage disease.
4. Early stages of cancer of the rectum, treated with preoperative chemo and radiotherapy, can cause complete regression of the cancer and in time with further improvements this may become the treatment of choice[41] and has already significantly reduced the need for major surgery.
5. Endovascular intervention by implanting stents has curtailed the necessity for open coronary artery bypass surgery.[42]
6. Vagotomy to treat peptic ulcer disease has been replaced by medical treatment.[43]
7. Open aortic aneurysms replacement with a graft is increasingly being replaced by endo-vascular stents.[44]
8. Bariatric surgery is increasingly being replaced by the temporary insertion of balloons into the stomach.[45]
9. Cancer of the anus was[46] treated exclusively by excision, with the necessity for a colostomy until the mid-1990s. The treatment of choice now is chemo-radiation, with surgery reserved for cancers not responsive to chemotherapy or when a recurrence occurs.
10. Endoscopic insertion of stents for inoperable carcinoma of the oesophagus[47] replace a laparotomy assisted placement of the stent.

4. The causes of operative morbidity and mortality.

Once anaesthesia was established in 1846, serious causes of post-operative morbidity and mortality became common for the first time. It took 100 years, during this fifth period, for these complications to be avoided or controlled by prophylaxis or treatment. These changes have led to significant improvement in the prognosis of patients undergoing surgery.

The first and greatest cause of post-operative mortality, going back to earliest antiquity, were infections of wounds following either surgery or violence, that frequently led to septicaemia and death. Other complications include haemorrhage, dehydration and deep vein thrombosis (DVT) the cause of pulmonary embolism. In addition, a non-life-threatening problem should also be considered. This was when surgeons undertaking abdominal operations had to contend with severe spasm of the abdominal muscles. This required strong assistants to hold the wound open while the surgeon was operating and also caused difficulties when closing the abdomen, the problem was only solved when muscle relaxants were introduced and could be properly calibrated.

Septicaemia was the commonest cause of post-operative death before Lister's anti-septic operating technique was introduced. It was the cause of the high mortality amongst the patients who had undergone the first hysterectomies as has already been mentioned. Another example of postoperative infection causing high mortality followed Professor Theodor Billroth's operation of total thyroidectomy.[48] This was an original operation in 1860, abandoned because the mortality from post-operative septicaemia had reached 40%.

In antiquity, the production of pus in wounds was considered part of the normal healing process, for when pus was absent foul dressings were often placed in the wound to stimulate 'laudable pus'. Dr Guido Majno[49] records that in ancient times it was thought 'Good for a wound to rot a little', and if not, then 'to put something into the wound that will get it to rot'. He considered this 'The most pernicious and persistent mistake in the history of surgery'. This belief in the necessity for pus as part of the healing process did not change until the germ theory of disease was proved in 1858.

For while the ancients encouraged the formation of pus, in more modern times no such encouragement has been needed, as pathogenic bacteria swarmed everywhere in the dirty and unhygienic cities and towns of Europe. In London, the repeated cholera epidemics between 1832 and 1866 claimed thousands of lives. These deaths can be used as a marker of the total lack of hygiene that then prevailed. Cholera is caused by people drinking water polluted by *Vibrio cholerae,* having leaked into the drinking water as raw sewage. These repeated epidemics precipitated the building of the first sewage and clean water provision that London had ever had and was only completed in 1875, less than 150 years ago.

Pasteur's discovery of the germ theory of disease published in 1858 inspired Professor Joseph Lister to develop his 'antiseptic technique of operating'. This was published in 1865 and was successful in significantly reducing the postoperative death rate. Box 13.4 gives a brief Timeline of the history of sepsis through the ages.

Box 13.4.

Sepsis through the ages.

c 180 AD. Galen noticed that the wounds of a small number of gladiators healed without infection. This information was forgotten or unnoticed.[50]

1257. Theodoric of Lucca[51] declared that, 'Pus is not laudable'. He was ignored.

1673. Bacteria were identified microscopically.[52]

1846. Empirical observation led Professor Semmelweis to insist on hand washing before entering his maternity ward in Vienna immediately after attending post-mortems. Deaths from puerperal sepsis were reduced from 19% to 1%.[53]

1858. Microorganisms and the germ theory of disease was confirmed by Louis Pasteur.[54]

1865. In direct response to Pasteur's findings, Lister developed an anti-septic process to kill air borne micro-organisms while operating.[55]

1879. Sir Robert Tait pioneered an aseptic technique for operating that is still the standard practice today.[56]

1899. Introduction of surgical gloves [57]

1929. The discovery of penicillin.[58]

1943. A million doses of penicillin accompany the allied invasion of Normandy.[59]

1967. Bacterial resistance to penicillin was first recognised. This is now a threat as antibiotics become less effective in preventing sepsis in surgical wounds when used prophylactically or inappropriately clinically.[60]

2015. The incidence of antibiotic resistance continues to increase. Resistant bacteria cause as many infections in Europe as flu, HIV and tuberculosis combined. In the UK in 2015–2016, there were over 16,000 cases. In the EU in 2015 33,000 died. This has followed the increased use of antibiotics not only for humans, but also routinely, in large quantities, for animal husbandry.[61]

The mass production of antibiotics from 1943 onwards made the second half of the 20th century the safest time in history to undergo an operation. It then seemed that sepsis was a scourge of the past and had been consigned to history. A crack in the armour appeared when in 1967 bacterial resistance to penicillin was first recognised.

By the 21st century, the number of deaths due to antibiotic resistant bacteria climbed to 33,000 recorded in the European Union in 2015. This underlines the urgent need for the development of new antibiotics. Development of bacterial resistance to antibiotics is a natural and striking example of evolution in action. In a suitable environment, bacteria can divide every ten to twenty minutes with changes in DNA, while we humans multiply approximately every twenty or so years. The bacteria have the advantage.

The next commonest cause of post-operative deaths was exsanguination. Haemorrhaging arteries were first ligated in the 1st century AD by Celsus[63] a technique that Galen later used, saving many gladiators from death. In the Early Middle Ages, this technique was unknown until the Greek treatises of Galen reached Europe.

In modern warfare, tourniquets are now incorporated into soldier's battle-dress, ready to be used to stop major arterial bleeding following severe wounds caused by an exploding land mine to the legs.

In the late 19th century, dehydration was beginning to be recognised as a significant cause of death, especially in patients suffering from obstruction of the gut, due to colonic cancer for example. Before anaesthetics were available these patients could not even be considered for surgery and all died from dehydration. This is caused by the continuing accumulation of the normal secretions that enter the gut to facilitate digestion, but as the fluid is not reabsorbed, the gut continues to distend, so losing more fluid from the circulation that could not be replaced until intra-venous infusions were available.[64]

On a separate note, blood loss by haemorrhage was first corrected by transfusion during the First World War.[65]

Another cause of sudden death that occurs a few days postoperatively is a massive pulmonary embolus, secondary to deep vein thrombosis. Deep vein thrombosis begins commonly in the leg and pelvic veins. To reduce the incidence of DVT, the following measures have been developed, anti-embolic stockings are used to exert a decreasing pressure gradient from the foot upwards, facilitating the flow of venous blood towards the heart. This has proved insufficient in preventing DVTs, so inflatable cuffs that compress the calves every 30 seconds were then wrapped round the lower leg during the course of the operation. This helped, but the most effective prophylactic against DVT was and is regular injections of heparin.[66] These measures between them have successfully reduced the incidence of DVT causing pulmonary embolus to being a rare complication.

Last in this group of post-operative complications were severe muscle spasms in patients under anaesthesia. Muscle relaxants were first used during surgery in 1942, the ability to calibrate the correct dose to only last for the length of each operation was not finalised for over twenty years. Once done, anaesthesia reached new levels of safety and patients then had the advantage of narcosis, analgesia and muscle relaxation during an operation.[67] All these measures were developed during the second half of the 20th century and have contributed significantly to the safety of surgery.

Box 13.5.

Numbers of original operations in the fifth period from 1846 to 1981.

USA	15.
UK of Gt Britain & Ireland.	15.
(England 11)	
(Scotland 3)	
(Ireland 1 before1937)	
Germany.	7.
France	4.
Austria	3.
Switzerland.	1.
Moravia.	1.
England or USA.	1.
Total	47.

5. Countries where original operations took place.

Box 13.5 gives the countries where original operations in the fifth period took place. Forty-seven operations developed during this comparatively short time of 135 years. All these original operations took place in Western Europe and the United States of America, with the exception of one in Moravia.

The United Kingdom and the USA both produced 15 operations, Germany seven, France four and Austria three. Switzerland produced one, as did Moravia. In the operation concerning surgery for babies with spina-bifida, it has not been possible to decide whether it was first carried out in the USA or the UK, hence it has been attributed to both. The overall distribution of original operations in this period divides approximately into a third each for the UK, USA and Continental Europe.

6. Technical advances that made surgery safer.

By the end of this fifth period, it became a reality that all the internal tissues and organs of the body had been operated upon. However, immediately following the wide availability of ether in 1846, surgeons seemed to stand back to take stock of what operations were now feasible. The ease of communication through medical journals and surgical conferences had gathered momentum and surgeons knew about Dr Ephraim McDowell's[68] successful abdominal operation of 1809. Here the gynaecologists had the lead and it is perhaps not surprising that the first major original operation under anaesthesia was a hysterectomy.

Box 13.6.

Twenty-one original operations that consisted of whole organ excisions that took place between 1853 and 1925.

Hysterectomy	1853[70]
Thyroidectomy	1860[71]
Splenectomy	1867[72]
Kidney excision	1869[73]
Laryngectomy	1873[74]
Oesophagectomy	1877[75]
Colectomy	1879[76]
Gastrectomy	1881[77]
Cholecystectomy	1882[78]
Excision of fallopian tube	1883[79]
Pneumonectomy	1895[80]
Appendicectomy	1887[81]
Excision of pituitary	1889[82]
Adrenalectomy	1889[83]
Acoustic neuroma	1894[84]
Prostatectomy	1904[85]
Excision of rectum	1907[86]
Pancreatectomy	1909[87]
Thymectomy	1912[88]
Excision of bladder	1918[89]
Parathyroidectomy	1925[90]

Some surgeons prepared themselves by testing operations on animals before carrying them out on patients. Examples include a successful gastrectomy on a dog by Professor Theodor Billroth[69] in 1881, then in 1950, Dr Richard Lawler carried out the first successful whole organ transplant of a kidney also by showing that the operation was successful in dogs.

Despite this approach, post-operative mortality was initially high, this gradually decreased, as surgical skills improved and each of the measures to secure safer operations, as previously mentioned were brought into play. In so doing this underlines the second half of the 20th century as the safest period in all history for patients to have an operation, this record is now under threat from antibiotic resistant bacteria.

7. Whole organ excisions dominated surgery at the start of this period.

During the seven years following the introduction of anaesthesia, it seemed that potential trailblazing surgeons were considering where they should start. What actually happened is shown in the Box 13.6, where it is clear that excisions of whole organs from the abdomen, thorax and head and neck was the surgical path that they followed.

Patients at that time presented to surgeons with gross and long-standing pathology. One example was of a patient with severe and recurrent pain from large kidney stones, that were so large that the surgeon could easily palpate them on physical examination. If the patient's other kidney was not affected, excision of the pathological kidney[73] would relieve that patient from much suffering.

Following this trend, the largest coherent group of original operations now took place during the next 72 years. Thirteen involved abdominal whole organ excisions, three intra-thoracic organ excisions and five head and neck organ excisions. Obviously, single organs and pairs of diseased organs could not be excised.

The surgical technique to excise each of these organs involves gaining safe access to them, the complexity of which varies with each operation, although the general principles for excision are the same. First, it was necessary to gain access to the target organ, then identify and ligate the supplying artery or arteries. This allowed the venous blood in the organ to drain out before ligating the veins to de-vascularise the organ. For example, a kidney has as a rule only one artery and one vein to be ligated. In addition, the ureter between the kidney and bladder must also be ligated and divided, then it must be separated from the adrenal gland, before the kidney could be removed.

In the case of resecting a portion of diseased gut, whether stomach, small bowel or colon, requires the blood vessels supplying it to be secured and following excision, an anastomosis must be carried out, either to restore continuity in the bowel, or form a stoma through the abdominal wall so faeces can be discharged and collected in a bag. By removing these organs, surgeons became familiar with the anatomy and surgery required and this knowledge together with necessary skills was passed on to their trainees.

8. The increasing complexity of surgery.

Box 13.7.
Abdominal operations of increasing complexity from 1871 to 1970.

Intussusception of the caecum.	1871[91]
Acute Appendicitis.	1877[81]
Surgery for liver failure.	1903[92]
Perforated gastric ulcer	1904[93]
Hiatus hernia and anti-reflux op	1906[94]
Pyloric stenosis in infants.	1907[95]
Vagotomy for peptic ulceration.	1943[96]
Bariatric surgery.	1953[97]
Reconstruction of the anus.	1969[98]
Gastrointestinal reconstructions.	1970[99]

Surgeons from 1871 were discovering a wider range of conditions and diseases that could be treated surgically, that for the first time either saved or prolonged life. These are listed in Box 13.7. The first of these was an operation on children who suffered an intussusception of the caecum.[91] A condition where the terminal ileum invaginates the caecum and obstructs the flow of the contents of the gut. Until intussusceptions were reduced surgically from 1871, the outcome was usually fatal.

Another condition was pyloric stenosis in babies where gross thickening of the muscle prevents food and liquids passing from the stomach into the duodenum.[95] Again before surgery was undertaken in 1901, this condition was usually fatal.

The next two conditions, if not operated on in a timely fashion, become infected by bacteria. Before operations were undertaken to treat them patients usually progressed to septicaemia with tragic consequences. The first of these was perforation of the stomach[93] or duodenum, where the base of a peptic ulcer gives way followed by acid and gas flowing into the peritoneal cavity causing severe pain and widespread peritonitis. The diagnosis can be made by examination alone, as the principle sign is 'abdominal rigidity', where the patient keeps very still with their abdominal muscles in spasm. Any movement exacerbates the already severe pain. The perforation is closed at operation by suturing a flap of the omentum over it to seal the defect. This simple procedure was and is effective.

The second operation in this category was acute appendicitis, first operated on in 1887. [100]This disease if neglected results in inflammation spreading within the peritoneal cavity. This can cause a localised abscess or peritonitis. When surgeons began to routinely operate on patients with acute appendicitis, they also had the opportunity to wash out the peritoneal cavity with an antiseptic if there was pus as this helped to prevent further infection.

It was also about this time surgeons began to insert drains into the peritoneal cavity through small skin incisions to enable any residual discharge or pus to drain out of the abdomen. This manoeuvre considerably reduced the risk of the patient developing a post-operative abscess if there was peritoneal contamination.

Sir Zachary Cope,[101] an eminent English surgeon, had been puzzled by the fact that perforations of gastric or duodenal ulcers were only operated on for the first time thirteen years after Professor Theodor Billroth had carried out the more complex operation of gastrectomy in 1881. In 1953, Cope wrote, 'that it seemed strange that surgeons had dared to carry out complicated operations on the stomach before they ventured to operate for abdominal conditions which were obvious matters of urgency'. The explanation was simply that patients with diseases within the abdominal cavity, complicated by sepsis, had nearly always died before the days of anaesthesia. These patients were now beginning to be successfully operated on as emergencies.

Another operation improved the quality of life in patients with a cirrhotic liver and first took place in 1903. This was a bypass to divert blood from the portal vein that carries blood directly from the gut to the liver,[92] by connecting it to the systemic venous system, in this case the inferior vena cava. This had the effect of lowering the pressure in the portal vein, so preventing severe venous haemorrhage into the stomach or oesophagus that carries a high mortality, due to the fragility of these distended veins. This shunt operation is now obsolete having been replaced by endoscopic and endovascular procedures. These new techniques improve the quality and longevity of life. However, the ultimate operation for these patients remains a liver transplant.[102]

Next was hiatus-hernia repair[94] first carried out in 1906. The operation aimed to prevent regurgitation of acid from the stomach into the oesophagus to prevent it from becoming chronically inflamed, a condition that over time can cause cancer. A more recent operation has been to construct a 'flutter valve' at the lower end of the oesophagus to prevent reflux.

Also, within this category was the operation of vagotomy, first performed in 1943.[96] Complete division of the vagal nerves stops all acid secretion in the stomach and enables duodenal ulcers to heal. This was a chronic disease, in England where it caused a million days of work to be lost due to ill health in

1953. This operation is now obsolete as duodenal ulcers are now successfully treated medically with antibiotics and acid secretion suppressors.

A new disease for surgeons' attention was and is morbid obesity, recognised at the beginning in the second half of the 20th century. It is diagnosed when an individual's body mass index (BMI) is nearly twice that expected for their height. Morbid obesity is confirmed if the person's BMI is over 45, when it should be 25 or less, or when they carry more than 50 kilos above their expected ideal body weight. The first bypass operation to defunction a greater portion of the small bowel was undertaken in 1953 and was successful in achieving weight loss.[97] Morbid obesity is now of epidemic proportions and has resulted in specialised bariatric surgical units being developed. Treatment is already beginning to move away from operating, to the insertion of a 'balloon' into the stomach, by way of the mouth, thereby reducing the sensation of hunger so the patient eats less and loses weight.

Box 13.8.

Developments in neurosurgery, orthopaedics and eye surgery between 1879 and 1981.

Excision of a brain tumour.	1879[103]
Development of spinal ops.	1883[104]
Internal fixation of fractures.	1892[105]
Missile wounds of brain treated.	1915[106]
Synthetic lens implant in the eye.	1950[107]
Closure of spina bifida.	1955[108]
Harrington's rods	1958[109]
Total hip replacement.	1961[110]
In utero foetal surgery	1981[111]

The final operations in this group were gastro-intestinal reconstructions.[99] These involve the construction of pouches fashioned from a loop of small bowel and used to replace the stomach, rectum or bladder following the total excision of these organs. A pouch to replace the rectum is usually for patients who have severe ulcerative colitis. The pouches for the stomach and bladder follow total excision of these organs for cancer. All of these operations demonstrate increasing sophistication and ingenuity in gastro-intestinal surgery.

9. Further development of original operations in this period.

Other original operations include the first excision of a brain tumour that was carried out in 1879.[103] By 1915, during the First World War, metal fragments were surgically extracted from the brain, sometimes with the aid of a magnet.[106]

In 1955, a new and complex problem affecting new born babies needed to be addressed. These were babies with myelomeningocele, a defect in the spine and spinal canal that fails to close before birth. In the past, these babies rapidly became infected and did not live. It was only when antibiotics became available after 1943 that these babies survived. They then needed the spinal defect to be closed and afterwards if they developed hydrocephalus to have a cerebro-peritoneal shunt inserted.[108] Because of the difficulties and complications of surgery in these seriously disabled babies, decisions concerning operating on them led to wide-ranging discussions of how this condition should be managed. This eventually led to 'Ethics Committees' being established in hospitals to discuss this and other difficult problems arising from both medicine and surgery.

One result was that intra-foetal surgery[111] began to be undertaken to close the myelomeningocele at the base of the spine before birth to try to improve the prognosis. This was first carried out in 1981 and has achieved some success. This complex operation carries risks for both mother and baby and is still under review.

Box 13.9.

Development of cardiac and peripheral vascular surgery from 1896 to 1948.

First arterial reconstruction	1896[112]
Repair of aortic aneurysm	1906[113]
Mitral valvotomy	1923[114]
Repair of Fallot's tetralogy	1943[115]
Vascular bypass surgery	1948[116]

Other entries for orthopaedic surgery include Harrington's rods,[109] which are attached to the spine to treat scoliosis. Then there were successful hip joint replacements,[110] all represent advanced and sophisticated original operations.

Cardiac and peripheral vascular surgery operations range from repairs to arteries,[112] following either trauma or disease see Box 13.9 to replacement of aortic and other aneurysms with synthetic grafts,[113] through to open heart surgery,[114] that includes repair of the severe congenital abnormality of Fallot's tetralagy[115] and also vascular bypass surgery.[116]

By the end of the 19th century, great satisfaction in the progress of surgery was expressed by Sir John Erichsen,[117] a surgeon who declared, 'We have carried the art of surgery to the highest degree of perfection of which as an art it is susceptible'. This was only the early days of internal surgery and Sir John would have marvelled at how surgery further progressed. He was only wrong in his timescale as it took another 100 years for the accomplishment of original operations on all the tissues and organs of the body to have been completed.

10. Transplant operations.

There have been claims that skin transplants were carried out by the Hindu surgeon Sushruta in about 200 BC. This appears unlikely, Sushruta clearly describes his plastic original operations used for ear-lobe and nose reconstructions.[118] There was no description of free skin grafting in his writings.

The earliest known transplant of skin and therefore an original operation was an autograft that took place in France in 1740 by Dr Garengeot[119] a French surgeon. The next recorded transplant was of a cornea[120] in Moravia in 1906.

These were followed by the first major organ transplant of a kidney carried out by Dr Richard M. Lawler[121] an American surgeon in 1954. The kidney he transplanted survived five years. This was remarkable as it was implanted before any anti-rejection treatment was available. He had prepared carefully and established beforehand that the operation was successful when practised on dogs. This was the first whole organ transplant and the generic original operation of all transplants that followed. All are complex operations and difficult undertakings in their own right. A total of eleven are described and presented in Addendum as successor operations for reasons that will be explained.

11. Summary.

During the 135 years of this fifth period, there were 47 generic original operations. These involved outstanding advances in operating technique made possible by the development of new technologies, including the use of anaesthesia along with the advantages of improved instruments, avoidance of many hazards of the past such as sepsis, dehydration and deep vein thrombosis and other advances.

The operations of this fifth period are also remarkable for demonstrating an overall steady increase in the complexity of surgery over time. It started with whole organ excisions and then as confidence and knowledge grew to undertake difficult operations designed to improve function. These included shunts to prevent the development of hydrocephalus, repair of hiatus hernias, many of the orthopaedic operations, cranial surgery and vascular replacement surgery to mention but a few.

This period also witnessed the first successful whole organ transplant of a kidney that was a generic original operation and its importance will be further discussed in the next chapter.

All these accomplishments confirm that surgery has reached a level of maturity and sophistication unimaginable a century before. If all the original operations of this fifth period are added to those of the first two, along with the handful from the fourth, medieval period, it becomes evident that all the tissues and organs of the body had been operated on and excised where possible by 1981. A process that has taken surgeons nearly12,000 years to accomplish.

The history of surgery has been an extraordinary achievement involving generations of surgeons in different countries and cultures. From the beginning there has been an extraordinary continuity of the craft that emerged from the remote magic of trephinations in Peru that spread across the Eurasian continents, to be practised by Hippocrates thousands of years later and is still practised today.

It was the Ancient Egyptians who laid the foundations of surgery. Later, Hippocrates developed a theory that provided a framework within which medicine and surgery were to be practised until the discovery of the true causes of disease was known in the 19th century.

For surgery itself, it was the Ancient Greeks and Romans, with a significant contribution from India, who produced the first golden age of surgery with an impressive number of original operations. In fact, because they had operated so extensively on the superficial tissues of the body, no further original operations were undertaken during the next 1,300 years.

This extraordinary long period with no original operations was made worse by the Edict of Tours in 1163 which delayed the development of surgery.

The standard and variety of surgery practised by the Ancient Greeks was finally matched and exceeded by the operations of John Hunter. The philosophy and framework for the practice of surgery as laid down by Hippocrates was finally dethroned when the actual causes of disease were discovered.

There is also no plausible evidence that any of the operations of the ancients were reinvented, for it was their written descriptions of these original operations that reached the west and slowly began to be practised again in the Middle Ages and resulted in a gradual renaissance of the operations of the Ancient Egyptians, Greeks, Romans and Indians.

The modern era of surgery following anaesthesia was the second golden age of surgery, with the largest number of original operations being undertaken.

The philosophy of the gradual surge of original operations in this fifth period was driven by the realisation that with anaesthesia all the organs and tissues of the body might be operated upon and was underpinned by the rise of science and technology. It also required a detailed grasp of anatomy, and an understanding of physiology, also the development of new surgical instruments and diagnostic tools, from x-rays to MRI scanners. This was accompanied by the steady increase in understanding the causes of diseases especially infection that so dominated surgery in the past. There was also the challenge of how to reduce post-operative complications, this has been achieved.

This rapid expansion of ever more sophisticated original operations took place in Western Europe and the United States of America, where technology rapidly advanced and surgery became available to the many and not just the few. Now the sheer volumes of operations carried out has increased to the extent that the United Kingdom's Nation Health Service is the largest organisation in the country with over a million employees. All these advances took place in less than a century and a half.

This brings to an end the undertaking of original operations for no more have been produced or found since 1981. However, we have not reached the end of the story.

References:

Note. References to Chapter 2, lead to The Index and Timeline, which gives a Chapter where the relevant article is to be found under the date of the original operation.

1. Mr Robert Liston. Wikipedia.
2. Chapter 2. 1846. Anaesthetics.
3. Ibid. 1853. Hysterectomy.
4. Ibid. 1881. First gastrectomy.
5. William Stewart Halstead. Cameron J.L., Ann. Surgery. 1999: 225: 445–458.
6. Selection of Individuals for Training in Surgery. Bann S., Darzi A. Am. J. Surg. 190 (2005): 98–102.

7. *The End of the Golden Age of General Surgery. 1870–2000.* by N.K. Maybury. Published by Amazon. 2014, p. 128.
8. *The End of the Golden Age of General Surgery. 1870–2000.* By N.K. Maybury. Published by Amazon. 2014, p 28.
9. Chapter 2. 1163. Edict of Tours.
10. Ibid. 1300. Barber-Surgeons Company.
11. Ibid. 1300. Surgical apprenticeships.
12. Ibid. 1768. Development of Teaching Hospitals in London.
13. Ibid. 1768. Examinations for surgeons.
14. Ibid. 1860. Foundation of Nightingale School of Nursing.
15. Ibid. 1881. Professor Theodor Billroth.
16. Ibid. 1881. Dr W.J. Halstead.
17. European Union Working Time Directive. https//www.gov.uk
18. Chapter 2. 1846. Introduction of anaesthesia.
19. Ibid. 1858. Discovery of microorganisms.
20. Ibid. 1865. Antiseptic operating technique.
21. Ibid. 1879. Introduction of electricity.
22. Ibid. 1895. Discovery of x-rays.
23. Ibid. 1896. Discovery of radiation.
24. Ibid. 1899. Intravenous fluids.
25. Ibid. 1908. Introduction of electro-diathermy.
26. Ibid. 1910. Introduction of laparoscopy.
27. Ibid. 1915. Blood transfusion.
28. Ibid. 1923. Angiography.
29. Ibid. 1929. Angioplasties and stenting of arteries.
30. Ibid. 1929. Discovery of Penicillin.
31. Ibid. 1935. Discovery of Heparin.
32. Ibid. 1940. Invention of ultrasound.
33. Ibid. 1958. Introduction of flexible endoscopy.
34. Ibid. 1994. CT scanners. And, The End of the Age of General Surgery. 1870–2000. N.K. Maybury. CreateSpace Independent Publishing Platform, North Charleston, South Carolina. 2014. p 35–37.
35. Chapter 2. 1998. Magnetic resonance scans.
36. Ibid. 2000. Robotic assisted operations.
37. Ibid. 1903 Cirrhosis of the liver.

38. The Changing Face of Surgery. An Inaugural Lecture by Sir Peter Bell delivered in the University of Leicester as Foundation Professor of Surgery, 29th October 1974. Published at the University of Leicester Press. 1975. p 16.
39. Chapter 2. 1860. Thyroidectomy.
40. Ibid. 1873. Laryngectomy.
41. Ibid. 1907. Treatment of rectal cancer.
42. Ibid. 1948. Coronary bypass operations.
43. Ibid. 1943. Vagotomy.
44. Ibid. 1906. Aortic aneurysm surgery.
45. Ibid. 1953. Bariatric surgery.
46. Cancer of the anus. analcancer.nhs.uk.
47. The End of the Golden Age of General Surgery. 1870–2000. by N.K. Maybury. Published by Amazon. 2014. pp 112–114. Oesophageal surgery.
48. Chapter 2. 1860. Thyroidectomy.
49. Dr Guido Majno. The Healing Hand. Harvard University Press. 1971, p 184.
50. Chapter 2. 180 AD. Galen.
51. Ibid. 1257. Theodoric of Lucca.
52. Ibid. 1673. Identification of bacteria.
53. Ibid. 1846. Professor Semmelweis.
54. Ibid. 1858. Germ theory of disease.
55. Ibid. 1865. Antiseptic method of operating.
56. Ibid. 1865. Aseptic technique of operating
57. Ibid. 1899. Introduction of surgical gloves.
58. Ibid. 1929. Discovery of penicillin.
59. Ibid. 1944. A million doses of penicillin. (Find in article in 1929).
60. *The End of the Golden Age of General Surgery*. By N.K. Maybury, Printed by Amazon. 2014. pp 101–102.
61. Chapter 2. 1967. Antibiotic resistant bacteria. (See under entry for 1929).
62. *Missing Microbes. How killing bacteria creates modern plagues.* Martin J. Blaser. One world Publications, England. 2015.
63. Chapter 2. c30 BC. Celsus.
64. Ibid. 1902. Introduction of intra-venous fluids.

65. Ibid. 1915. Blood transfusion
66. Ibid. 1936. Discovery of Heparin.
67. Ibid. 1942. Introduction of muscle relaxants. (Find in article under entry for 1846).
68. Ibid. Dr Ephraim McDowell
69. Ibid. 1881. Professor Theodor Billroth.
70. Ibid. 1853. Hysterectomy.
71. Ibid. 1860. Thyroidectomy.
72. Ibid. 1867. Splenectomy.
73. Ibid. 1869. Excision of kidney.
74. Ibid. 1873. Laryngectomy.
75. Ibid. 1877. Oesophagectomy.
76. Ibid. 1879. Colectomy.
77. Ibid. 1881. Gastrectomy.
78. Ibid. 1882. Cholecystectomy.
79. Ibid. 1883. Salpingectomy for ectopic pregnancy.
80. Ibid. 1895. Pneumonectomy.
81. Ibid. 1887. Appendicectomy.
82. Ibid. 1889. Excision of pituitary.
83. Ibid. 1889. Adrenalectomy.
84. Ibid. 1894. Acoustic neuroma.
85. Ibid. 1904. Prostatectomy.
86. Ibid. 1907. Excision of rectum.
87. Ibid. 1909. Pancreatectomy.
88. Ibid. 1912. Thymectomy.
89. Ibid. 1918. Excision of bladder.
90. Ibid. 1925. Parathyroidectomy.
91. Ibid. 1871. Intussusception of caecum.
92. Ibid. 1903. Surgery for liver failure.
93. Ibid. 1892. Perforated gastric ulcer.
94. Ibid. 1919. Hiatus hernia repair.
95. Ibid. 1907. Ramstedt's operation, pyloric stenosis.
96. Ibid. 1943. Vagotomy.
97. Ibid. 1953. Bariatric surgery.
98. Ibid. 1969. Anal reconstruction.
99. Ibid. 1969. Reconstructive gut surgery.

100. Ibid. 1887. Acute appendicitis.
101. Sir Zachary Cope. *Seventy Years of Abdominal Surgery. Science Medicine and History, Essays on the evolution of scientific thought and medical practice. Volume Two*. Edited by E. Ashworth Underwood. Oxford University Press, 1953, p 341.
102. Chapter 2. 1903. Surgery for liver failure.
103. Ibid. 1879. Excision of brain tumour.
104. Ibid. 1883. Spinal operations.
105. Ibid. 1892. Internal fixation of fractures.
106. Ibid. 1915. Intracranial surgery for missile injuries.
107. Ibid. 1950. Implant of synthetic intraocular lens.
108. Ibid. 1955. Cerebral-peritoneal shunts for hydrocephalus.
109. Ibid. 1958. Harrington's rods.
110. Ibid. 1961. Total Hip replacement.
111. Ibid. 1981. In utero foetal surgery.
112. Ibid. 1896. First arterial reconstruction.
113. Ibid. 1906. First repair of aortic aneurysm.
114. Ibid. 1923. Mitral valvotomy.
115. Ibid. 1943. Operations for Fallot's tetralogy.
116. Ibid. 1948. Vascular bypass surgery.
117. Sir John Erichsen. Brit Med. Journal, 1873, ii, 414–415.
118. Chapter 2. .c200 BC. Sushruta's plastic surgery.
119. Ibid. 1740. Skin, the first transplant of skin.
120. Ibid. 1906. Corneal transplant.
121. Ibid. 1950. Kidney transplant.

Chapter 14

The End of an Era of Surgery

The identification of original operations, as described in Chapter 1, is complete. The inclusion of the following eleven complex transplants, although not technically original operations, they are vital additions to complete a 'First Era of Surgery,' when all the 'Tissues and organs of the body have been operated upon, excised and transplanted where possible'.

Box 14.1.

Increasing complexity of transplant operations following the kidney transplant of 1950. These are not classified as original operation.

1. 1963 Liver transplant.[4]
2. 1963 Heart transplant.[5]
3. 1966 Pancreatic transplant.[6]
4. 1983 Lung transplant.[7]
5. 1987 Liver/heart and lung transplant.[8]
6. 1993 Thymus transplant.[9]
7. 2000 Hand transplant.[10]
8. 2005 Face transplant.[11]
9. 2012 Arm transplant.[12]
10. 2014 Transplant of uterus.[13]
11. 2018 Penile transplant.[14]

The meticulous organisation and complex surgery necessary to undertake these eleven transplants is recognised in this book. It has been of great personal interest for the author, as a surgeon himself, to closely follow their success, as they are an integral part of this history.

To continue, the first known transplant was of the skin[1] in 1740. Followed by a corneal[2] transplant in 1906. The next was the first whole organ transplant of a kidney[3] in 1950. Each were very different procedures and each is an original operation.

The kidney, in 1950, was the first whole organ to be transplanted and was the generic original operation of all the subsequent organ transplants that took place during the 45 years between 1963 and 2018 as shown in Box 14. 1

All whole organ transplants have fundamental anatomical similarities, these must be taken into account when operating. All need the careful removal of the diseased organ or limb from the transplant recipient. The viability of the organ to be transplanted follows the same pattern and depends on re-establishing the arterial blood inflow and venous outflow. Then with every organ other vital structures must be connected to restore the function of the whole organ.

For a transplanted kidney, the ureter must be implanted into the bladder. Following liver transplantation, the portal vein and common bile duct need to be appropriately anastomosed. In pancreatic transplants, the exocrine secretions must be drained into the gut. With limb transplants, nerves, tendons and muscles need to be connected.

So, for all their differences and complexity, it is the overall similarity in the operating process, that applies to the kidney transplant and these eleven successor transplants described in this chapter. It is this similarity, while accepting that all were surgical triumphs, that means they cannot be included as original operations.

Ten of the 11 transplants follow the pattern described above. The odd one out is the thymus gland that is sliced and transplanted into muscle.

Transplant surgery has been so comprehensive that it now seems unlikely that there will be any new transplants, this makes it reasonable to believe that a seminal point in the history of surgery has now been passed, when all the tissues and organs of the body have been successfully operated upon, excised and transplanted where possible.

The comprehensiveness of all these operations is such that I believe it would now be correct to name the period from 10,000 BC to 2018 AD as the 'First Era of Surgery'.

1. Summary

This 'Unfamiliar History' has created a new perspective in understanding the development of surgery. By adding the tentative beginnings of surgery in Ancient Egypt, with the major contributions by the Ancient Greeks and Romans and a significant input from India together produced a substantial number of original operations on the superficial tissues of the body. The extent of this was so comprehensive that it was one reason why the Byzantines, Arabians and surgeons in Western Europe in the Middle Ages, until 1575, were unable to add any original operations. Throughout this lapse of 1300 years, surgeons did continue to undertake some of the operations of the ancients. Surgery in Western Europe had also been significantly retarded by the Edict of Tours of 1163, needing 700 years for the problems it caused to be erased,before surgeons were again on an equal footing with university trained physicians.

The beginning of science began in the 13th and 14th centuries and gradually lead to major improvements in technology. Amongst the subsequent discoveries was the use of Ether, that literally enabled the great cavities of the body to undergo planned surgery for the first time.

Going back, the continuity of surgery through different countries and empires over hundreds of years has been established. This was made possible by the written works of the Ancient Egyptians Greeks and Indians being translated through different languages, and the pathway of this transfer has been described in some detail. The modern fifth period produced the largest number of complex operations in under 150 years following which all the tissues and organs of the body have been operated upon and transplanted when possible. The Greek influence is now largely forgotten but still exists in the background when modern surgeons practise the common operations on the superficial tissues of the body. Surgeons are already advancing into a new technological and complex era. So, after the last original operation was carried out in 1981 and the last transplant in 2018 a definitive 'First Era of Surgery' has been identified. This is the end of the beginning for surgeons are already working with more sophisticated technology at the beginning of a second 'Era of Surgery'.

Dr William Harvey was right, when in 1627, he published his proof of the circulation of the blood and wrote, 'All new learning is built on that of those who have gone before'.

References:

1. Chapter 2, 1740. First skin transplant, an original operation.
2. Ibid. 1906. First corneal transplant, an original operation.
3. Ibid 2. 1950. First Kidney transplant, an original operation.
4. Addenda, 1963 Liver transplant.
5. Ibid. 1963 Heart transplant.
6. Ibid. 1966 Pancreatic transplant.

7. Ibid. 1983 Lung transplant.
8. Ibid. 1987 Liver/heart and lung transplant.
9. Ibid. 1993 Thymus transplant.
10. Ibid. 2000 Hand transplant.
11. Ibid. 2005 Face transplant.
12. Ibid. 2012 Arm transplant.
13. Ibid. 2014 Transplant of uterus.
14. Ibid. 2018 Penile transplant.

Addendum

The History and Descriptions of the Last Eleven Transplant Operations

1963. South Africa. First heart transplant.

The first heart transplant was by Dr Christiaan Barnard (1922–2001), a cardiac surgeon at the University of Cape Town. The patient died of pneumonia 18 days post-operatively. This was not due to failure of his heart transplant.[1] By 2011, the survival of heart and heart and lung transplants was approximately 70% at three years.[2]

References:

1. Wikipedia. Christiaan Barnard.
2. *General Surgery Lecture Notes* by Harold Ellis, Sir Roy Calne and Christopher Watson. Wiley-Blackwell 2011.

1963. USA. First liver transplant.

A liver transplant was first carried out by Dr Thomas Starzl (1927–2017) of Denver in the USA. Although technically successful it was not until 1967 that a patient survived for a year.[1] This was due to the introduction of cyclosporine, an immunosuppressant drug discovered in 1986 and introduced by Sir Roy Calne (1930–), Professor of Surgery at Cambridge, England. As a result, in the 1980s, the survival time following liver transplantation climbed to 85% at one year and by 2011, the five-year survival was around 70%.[2]

References:

1. Wikipedia. Thomas Starzl.
2. *General Surgery Lecture Notes* by Harold Ellis, Sir Roy Calne and Christopher Watson. Wiley-Blackwell 2011

1966. USA. First pancreatic transplant.

The first transplant of a whole pancreas was in Minnesota in the USA in 1966. The operation was successful and was published in 1967 by Dr W.D. Kelly *et al.,*[1] unfortunately the patient only survived three months to die from a massive pulmonary embolus.[2]

By 2010 in the USA, there had been 22,000 pancreatic transplants to treat the complications of diabetes mellitus. Following transplantation, these patients had no further need for insulin injections and their overall wellbeing was greatly enhanced with a better quality and length of life.

A few diabetic patients with related kidney failure received a kidney transplant alone, though this did not change their diabetic status. As transplants were proving successful, the majority of patients then underwent unrelated transplants of both the pancreas and duodenum, along with a kidney. The kidney was necessary due to diabetic induced renal failure. The donors were usually patients who had suffered a severe stroke or head injury, while occasionally a living donor gave their distal pancreas and a kidney.

The surgical technique involves taking the pancreas in a block with the duodenum. The ends of the duodenum are closed and the transplant placed on the right-hand side of the recipient's pelvis, a small bowel loop (roux-en-y) is then anastomosed to the donor's duodenum to allow the exocrine output of their implanted pancreas to flow into the recipient's small bowel. The kidney is placed in the left side of the pelvis outside the peritoneum to facilitate biopsies to monitor signs of rejection.

Transplanting pancreatic islet cells by injection into the liver began in the 1960s and by 2004, the number of patients with type 1 diabetes who received such implantation was 471. Of these 58% were insulin independent 12 months after implantation.

Allotransplantation of pancreas and duodenum along with kidney due to diabetic nephrology.

References:

1. Kelly W.D., Lillehei, R.C, Merkel, F.D., Idezuki, Y. & Goetz F.C Surgery. 1967. 61: 827–837. 15, Section 4.
2. Ricordi automated method of islet isolation. Piemont L., Pileggi A., 2013. CellR4. 1(1): 8–22.

1983. Canada. First successful lung transplant.

In 1983, Professor Joel D. Cooper carried out the first successful lung transplant at Toronto General Hospital in Canada. He was a graduate of Harvard Medical School. There had been many failed attempts by other surgeons before this. He also was the first to carry out a bilateral lung transplant.

Minimally invasive thoracic surgery was introduced in 1992. The uptake of this approach to thoracic surgery was initially slow. In the UK, video-assisted thoracoscopic surgery has increased to 50% of operations in recent years. Cooper considered that minimally invasive thoracic surgery would lead to a golden age, when very early diagnosis of lung cancer would result in surgery being limited to minor excisions through a minimally invasive approach, followed by adjuvant chemotherapy.

In the 1980s, he also studied the cause of ulceration of the trachea following intubation and developed a low-pressure endotracheal tube, the prototype of those used today.

Reference.

MedTech. Volume 01 Issue 02. January 2019. www.rcseng.ac.uk*1984.*

1984. England & USA. The Visualisation of internal organs by computerised tomography.

Computerised Tomography, CT, was invented in 1982 by Sir Godfrey Newbold Hounsfield (1919–2004) of EMI laboratories in England and Dr Allan MacLeod Cormac (1924–1998) of Tufts University, USA. Both were awarded the Nobel Prize for Peace in 1989 for their contribution to medicine and science.

The first clinical CT scanner was to image the head and many were installed in hospitals between 1984 and 1986. Then in 1990, whole-body scanners became available and were immediately pressed into service. The speed and resolution of the CT scanners has continued to improve over the years. Tomography works by sending multiple x-ray beams through the body at different angles. Detectors record how each beam passes through the body and a computer analyses these measurements to construct an internal image of the body, the result is then projected onto a screen.[1]

A good example of the clinical usefulness of CT head scans is to accurately identify haemorrhage and or oedema in the brain of patients with head injuries. Previously, the diagnosis of these injuries was purely on clinical grounds. In those days, patients suspected of having localised haemorrhage causing pressure on the brain, required emergency trephination of the skull to evacuate any haematoma and elevate depressed fractures if present. These patients were usually unconscious on arrival at an Accident & Emergency department.

Before CT scans were available, head injuries had to be diagnosed from the patient's history, gleaned from relatives or the ambulance crew, followed by a general examination to identify any other injuries and a detailed neurological examination. If it was uncertain whether trephination of the skull would be helpful or not, then exploratory burr-holes were carried out to ensure that no patient was denied treatment that might be lifesaving.

When computerised tomography became available, damage to the brain could now be visualised. If the scan showed gross oedema or brain damage, then surgical exploration was useless and no longer indicated. If a blood clot on the brain was identified, then surgery was immediately carried out. The CT scan had the added advantage that only a single burr-hole correctly placed might be all that was needed.

Before the availability of CT scans, surgeons had of necessity a low threshold to operating if there was any doubt. This became no longer necessary and it was reassuring to know that in the days when the diagnosis was entirely clinical, when the only investigation available was a plain an x-ray, that no one who might benefit from trephination had been missed.[2] The result was that the scans reduced the numbers of operations formerly carried out for head injuries.

References:

1. Science Museum on line. Techniques and Technologies. Ct/CAT scanner.

2. The End of the Golden Age of General Surgery, N.K. Maybury. CreateSpace Amazon. 2014. ISBN 1499531370. 78–80.

1984.England. Chemo-radiation treatment for carcinoma of the anus.

Until 1984, there was no known efficacious adjuvant treatment for squamous cell carcinoma of the anus. The standard treatment was an abdominoperineal excision of the anus, lower rectum and associated lymph nodes and resulted in the patient having a permanent colostomy. In addition, block dissections of the inguinal lymph nodes may be necessary as lymph from the anus drains into them.

A trial of giving preoperative radiotherapy with 5-Flouro-Uracil and a single dose of Mitomycin was carried out in a few patients. A few weeks after this treatment, they underwent planned abdominoperineal excisions of the anus. Subsequent histological examination found no signs of residual cancer at the time of their operation.[1] This led to a wait and see policy after radio and chemotherapy. By the middle of the 1980s, chemo radiation was becoming the treatment of choice for cancer of the anus, surgery being reserved for those patients who did not respond or subsequently developed recurrent disease.[2] This is an example of surgical treatment that may in time become obsolete.

References:

1. Dis. Colon Rectum 1984; 17:354–356.
2. Prognostic Factors for Squamous Cell Cancer of the Annual Canal. Gastrointest. Cancer Res. 2008 Jan–Feb: 2(1): 10–14.

1987. England. Cluster transplants of liver, heart and lung and others.

Sir Roy Calne (1930–), Professor of Surgery at Cambridge University was the first to carry out a combined, heart, liver and lungs transplant. He was also the first to identify immunosuppressive agents to prevent rejection of transplanted organs.

In 1994, he transplanted a combined cluster of organs into a patient that consisted of the stomach, intestine, pancreas, liver and one kidney. Also, in a patient with cystic fibrosis who needed transplants of both lungs, Calne found it technically simpler to transplant the lungs and the heart from a donor together. This meant that the heart of a patient with cystic fibrosis, which is usually healthy, could in turn be used as a donor organ. A similar process can be initiated in other cluster grafts to optimise the use of organs.[1]

'Cyclosporin' was the first active agent to be used for immune suppression in patients receiving donor grafts and was introduced by Professor Calne. Side effects caused by this drug are common and include increased susceptibility to bacterial and viral infections, high blood pressure and decreased kidney function[2] on the one hand, while on the other hand, it has enabled many thousands of patients to undergo successful organ transplants that with careful management are long lasting.

Heart-lung transplantation for cystic fibrosis and subsequent domino heart transplantation.

References:

1. Yacoub, M.H. *et al.,* The Journal of Heart Transplantation. (5): 459–466; discussion 466–7.
2. Organ Transplantation by Petechuk, David. Greenwood Press, Westport, USA. 2006. ISBN 0-313-33542-7.

1987. USA. Magnetic resonance imaging (MRI).

The first human MRI scan was in July 1987 when Dr Raymond Damadian (1936–) used a scanner he had built by hand at New York's Downstate Medical Centre. The science was to use nuclear magnetic resonance to create images of living tissue.

In 1937, Professor Isidor Isaac Rabi (1898–1988), a Professor at Colombia University, New York, recognised that atomic nuclei show their presence by absorbing or emitting radio waves when exposed to a sufficiently strong magnetic field. For this, he received the Nobel Prize for Physics in 1944. An MRI image is reconstructed from harmless radio waves emitted by a living organism and gives it an advantage over a CT scan that uses ionising radiation. MRI produces a steady magnetic field round the patient. Then the body is stimulated by radio waves to change the steady state orientation of protons. When the radio waves are turned off, the machine records the body's electromagnetic transmission to construct an internal image of the body.[1]

In the UK, there were 467 MRI scanners in 2014, at that date the UK had fewer per head of population than any other developed country. The machines are particularly used by neurologists, urologists and orthopaedic surgeons and now increasingly to diagnose thoracic and intra-abdominal disease.

Reference:

A short history of Magnetic Resonance Imaging (MRI). Tesla Memorial Society of New York. www.teslasociety.com.

1993. USA. Transplant of thymus gland.

Transplants of normal thymus glands began in 1993, with a total of 54 infants being treated by 2006. This series was published by Dr M.L. Markert *et al.,* in 2007.[1]

Thymus malfunction is caused by an A22q11 micro-deletion that is responsible variably, for thymic hypoplasia, cardiac malformations, craniofacial anomalies, cleft palate and hypothyroidism.[2] Other anomalies can include anal atresia, growth or developmental retardation, genital hypoplasia and deafness.[2]

The donors are children undergoing surgery for inherited cardiac defects, in whom the thymus is excised to allow access to the heart. These glands are then transplanted by implanting slices of them into the quadriceps muscle of the recipient by an open operation under general anaesthesia.

The results in 44 patients who received thymus transplants were successful in that they became euthymic and 64% of them survived. The 11 deaths were unrelated to the thymic transplant.[3]

Review of 54 patients with complete DiGeorge anomaly. Enrolled in protocols for thymus transplantation; Outcome of 44 consecutive thymus transplants.

References:

1. Markert M.L., Devlin B.H., Alexieff M.J., *et al.,* Blood. 2007 May 15: 109(10): 4539–3447.
2. Iris coloboma and a microdeletion of chromosome 22: del (22) (q11.22). D.A. Morrison, D.R. Fitzpatrick and B.W. Fleck. Br J Opthalmol. 2002 Nov: 86(11): 1316.
3. Chapter 2. See entry for 1912.

2000. Implementation of the European Union's Working Time Directive

Professor Theodor Billroth was arguably the greatest surgeon at the end of the 19th century and had also trained a generation of outstanding surgeons. Among them was Dr William S. Halstead[1] who returned to his native America and instituted a surgical residency programme in his hospital for trainee surgeons. This involved working under the supervision of consultant surgeons in a progression of appointments of increasing responsibility. This system was adopted in the United Kingdom and represented a modern form of apprenticeship.

This system of training was finally brought to an end in the UK by the European Union's working time directive in 2000.[2] The unintended consequence for surgery was the necessity for doctors to work in shifts to provide 24 hours cover every day of the year in hospitals, while keeping within the limits of the 48-hour working week. This short and inflexible week irrevocably changed the practice of surgery and the training of surgeons.

The result for trainee surgeons was the loss of the apprenticeship and close contact with consultant surgeons that had been the norm before the Working-Time Directive was implemented. Trainees had formerly worked under the supervision of their chief in outpatient and operating theatre sessions and attended ward-rounds regularly. Under the new system, consultants were now replaced by specialists, for instance a general and vascular surgeon from before the turn of the 21st century was replaced by an upper gut surgeon, a colonic surgeon, a liver and pancreas surgeon and a vascular surgeon. There was of course be some variation in this, but in addition the time taken to train the next generation of surgeons has been reduced from 80,000 hours to 10,000 hours.[3] How surgery was practiced at the end of the 20th century before these changes took place has been described by the author.[4] as this is now history.

References:

1. William Stewart Halstead. By Cameron J.L. Ann. Surgery. 1998; 225: 445–458.
2. *The End of the Golden Age of General Surgery 1870–2000. The Training and Practise of a General Surgeon in the late Twentieth Century.* By

Nigel Keith Maybury. Amazon Independent Publishing Platform 2014, ISBN: 1499531370. 128–131.
3. Bann, S. and Darzi, A. Selection for Individuals for Training in Surgery. Am. J. Surg. 190(2005): 98–102.
4. *The End of the Golden Age of General Surgery.* By N K Maybury. Amazon. 2014.

2000. USA. Robot assisted operations.

UJBI site.[1]

In the second decade of the twenty-first century, robotic operating systems were dominated by 'DaVinci', a company licenced in the USA in 2000. The DaVinci surgical robots are manufactured to operate through the same small ports used in non-invasive surgery. The use of robotics is more sophisticated than the same operation carried out through a laparotomy incision. Operations performed by using these instruments are not therefore original operations, but it is an impressive new technology to carry out already established operations.

The outcomes of robot assisted surgery were studied across a broad range of operations between 2000 and 2001. These included: 69 anti-reflux operations, 36 cholecystectomies, 26 Heller's myotomies, 17 bowel resections, 15 donor nephrectomies, 14 left internal mammary artery mobilisations, 7 gastric bypass operations, 7 splenectomies, 6 adrenalectomies, 3 exploratory laparoscopies, 4 pyloroplasties, 2 gastrojejunostomies, 1 distal pancreatectomy, one duodenal polypectomy, one gastrectomy, one esophagectomy and one lysis of adhesions.

There were three technical problems when the DaVinci system malfunctioned. These required conversion to standard laparoscopic operation. There were also 19 (4%) medical or surgical complications. Six were considered major and there was one death that was unrelated to the robotics. Since then, robotic assisted surgery has increased[2] significantly and spread widely throughout the world.

In 2010, a comparison was made between excising the rectum laparoscopically or by a robotically assisted operation. The outcomes were similar.[3] Surgery for papillary thyroid carcinomas and some cardiac operations appear difficult when undertaken robotically and appear to have been pursued with a view to maximising the cosmetic effect of the operation. Owing to complications, cardiac surgeons are now more cautious concerning robotic assisted surgery.[4]

The cost of robotic surgery is high; the machine costs approximately $2,000,000 in 2017. Some of the attachments are disposable. This increases the price of each operation by $3000 to $6000 more than a laparoscopic operation. In addition, 100,000 dollars are needed annually for parts and servicing costs.

Despite the cost, the operation of choice in the USA for carcinoma of the prostate is robot assisted. Patients lose less blood and the dissection of the organ is impressive, but the measurements of impotence and incontinence appear to be no better than open surgery.[5] In addition, the anastomosis of the urethra to the bladder with robotic aided surgery still appears difficult.

Time will identify the operations in which DaVinci robots produce superior surgical results. It is still too soon to call time on laparoscopic and open surgery. In the UK, as of May 2016, there were estimated to be only 60 robotic systems in use in the UK, so only one out of four major hospitals have this equipment and this indicates that the cost may limit the expansion of robotic surgery. It is possible that its considerable costs, including the time to carry out an operation, may become untenable if the results are not significantly superior.

References:

1. From Leonardo to da Vinci: the history of robot assisted surgery in urology. David R. Yates, Christophe Vaessen and Morgan Roupret. BJUI Academic Urology Department, la Piete-Salpetiere Hospital, Paris. And, Surgical Endoscopy and other Interventional techniques. M.A. Talmini, S. Chapman, S. Horgan, W.S. Melvin. Nature. Oct 2003, Vol. 17, Issue 10, pp 1521–1524.
2. Robotic-assisted versus laparoscopic surgery for low rectal cancer. Jun Seok Park *et al.,*
3. Annals of Surgical Oncology. Dec2010, Vol. 17, Issue 12. 3195–3202.
4. Robot assisted endoscopic surgery for thyroid cancer. Sang-Wook Kang *et al.,* Surgical Endoscopy. Nov 2009, 23: 2399.
5. New technology and healthcare costs. The case for robotic-assisted surgery. The New England Journal of Medicine. Gabriel I. Barbash, Sherry A. Gilied. 2010: 363; 701–704.

6. Is da Vinci Robotic Surgery a Revolution or rip off, by Cameron Scott, 2016.

2000. USA. Hand transplants.

Twenty-five hand transplants were carried out between 2000 and 2005. These are difficult transplants with the operations taking between eight and twelve hours, involving, re-establishing the circulation, bone fixation and anastomoses of the tendons and nerves.

Reference.

Organ Transplantation by David Petechuk. Greenwood Press, London 2006. ISBN 0-313-333542-7.

2005. France. First face transplant.

In November 2005, Dr Bernard Devauchelle and Dr Jean-Michel Dubernard in Amiens, France, performed the first elective partial face transplant on a 46-year-old woman who was given new cheeks, nose, chin and mouth following a devastating attack by a dog. Eighteen months later, she was satisfied with the result.[1]

The first full facial face transplant was in Barcelona in Spain in 2010. Five years after a farmer had accidentally shot himself, he underwent a 24 hours operation to give him a new face. The transplant included a jaw, cheekbones, muscles and eyelids.[1&2]

On the 15th August 2005, two months before the French face transplant, an auto-transplant was carried out on a nine-year-old Indian girl. Her face and scalp were amputated when her hair was caught in a threshing machine. The parents took their daughter to hospital with her face in a plastic bag. The surgeon managed to reconnect the arteries and replant the skin. The operation was successful but the patient was left, not surprisingly, with some muscle damage as well as scarring round the edge of the re-implant.[3]

References:

1. Organ Transplantation by David Petechuk. Greenwood press, Westport, London, 2006. ISBN 0-313-33542-7. 67.

2. The Guardian newspaper. https://www.thegardien.com/mar/face.
3. Wikipedia. History of face implant.

2012. USA. First bilateral arm transplants.

First bilateral arm transplant in the USA was by Dr W. P. Andrew Lee, Dr Richard Redett , Dr D. Cooney and Dr Gerald Brandacher of the Johns Hopkins Plastic and Reconstructive Surgery Unit.

Reference:

Johns Hopkins Medicine. First Ever Penis and Scrotum Transplant Makes History. Hopkinsmedicine.org by Karen Nitkin on 23/04/2018.

2014. Sweden. Uterine transplant followed by pregnancy and delivery of a healthy baby.

In 2014, a healthy baby was born to a uterine transplant recipient in Sweden. The uterus was from a 61-year-old donor and the recipient was 36. The surgical team was led by Dr Mats Brannstrom, Professor of Obstetrics and Gynaecology at the University of Gothenburg. The recipient was born with healthy ovaries but without a uterus. Immuno-suppression was successful using tacrolimus, azothiaprine and corticosteroids. The transplant was considered temporary and a hysterectomy is planned after one or two successful births.[1]

The first attempted uterus transplant was in 1931 in Germany. The recipient died from organ rejection three months later. Without a child being born, this transplant was unsuccessful and therefore not an original operation.

In 2011, Dr Munire Erman Akar transplanted a uterus from a deceased donor. The operation was a success, it is unknown if a successful birth followed. There have also been successful transplants in India and Brazil in 2017.

There is an ongoing debate concerning the ethics of this operation.

Reference:

Wikipedia. Uterus transplantation.

2018. USA. Penile transplant:

In 2018, a penile and scrotal transplant was carried out in USA by Dr W. P. Andrew Lee, Dr Richard Redett, Dr D. Cooney and Dr Gerald Brandacher. Testes were not transplanted as sperm would not be that of the recipient. Two weeks post-surgery the recipient received bone marrow infusions from the donor. This is a treatment pioneered at Johns Hopkins University to modulate the immune response with the result that patients only need low doses of immune suppression medication.[1]

Reference:

Johns Hopkins Medicine. First Ever Penis and Scrotum Transplant Makes History. Hopkinsmedicine.org by Karen Nitkin on 23/04/2018.

Bibliography

Allbutt, Thomas Clifford. *The Historical Relations of Medicine and Surgery to the End of the Sixteenth Century. An Address delivered at the St. Louis Congress in 1904.* London Macmillan and Co. 1905.

Arderne, Master John. *De Arte Phisicali et de Cirurgie.* Dated 1412. Translated by Sir D'Arcy Power from a transcript made by Edward Miller. Publishers, John Bale, Sons & Danielson, Ltd. Oxford Street, London, 1922. Hardpress, ISBN 0781407668208, www. hardpress.net.

Aristotle: The Complete Works. Aristotle. Kindle Edition, 2018.

Aristotle. Historia Animalium Vol. IV. The Works of Aristotle Translated into English, by D'Arcy Wentworth Thompson. 1910, Oxford at the Clarendon Press.

Aristotle. On Longevity and Shortness of Life. Kindle Edition, 2015.

Aristotle. On the Parts of Animals. Translated by William Ogle. Kessinger Publishing.

Avicenna. *The Canon of Medicine.* Adapted by Laleh Bakhtiar from the translations by O. Cameron Gruner and Mazar H. Shar, correlated with the Arabic by J.R. Crook. Great Books of the Islamic World, Inc. 1999. ISBN: 1-871031-67-2.

Bacci, Massimo Livi. *Our Shrinking Planet.* Translated by David Broder. Polity. English Edition 2017.

Bacon, Francis. Essays. Everyman. Edited by Michael J. Hawkins J.M. Dent, London. Reprinted 1999. ISBN: 0-460-874330.

Bacon, Roger. Medieval Philosophy: A Practical Guide to Roger Bacon. By M. James Ziccardi. ISBN 13: 978-14664 18325.

Bailey, Cyril, Editor. *The Legacy of Rome.* Oxford University Press. 1923, reprinted 1940.

Ball, James Moores. *Andreas Vesalius, The Reformer of Anatomy.* Trieste Publishing Facsimle printed 1910.

Bell, Professor Sir Peter.
The Changing Face of Surgery. An Inaugural Lecture. Leicester University Press 1975.

Bishop, W.J. Knife Fire and Burning Oil. 1960. Published by Robert Hale Ltd, London. ISNN 978-0-7090-9155-4.

Blaser, Martin. *Missing Microbes. How killing bacteria creates modern plagues.* One World Publications 1914.

Bhishagratna, Kaviraj Kunja Lal. *The Sushruta Samhita,* an English Translation. Volume 111. Published by S.L. Bhaduri, 10 Kashi Ghose's Lane, Calcutta. 1916.

Brock, Arthur J. *Greek Medicine. Being Extracts illustrative of Medical Writers from Hippocrates to Galen.* Editor Ernest Barker. J.M. Dent and Sons Ltd. London. 1929.

Cambridge Illustrated History of the World's Science. Colin A. Ronan. Book Club Associates London. The Press Syndicate of the University of Cambridge, 1983.

Campbell, Donald. *Arabian medicine and its Influence on the Middle Ages.* Volumes 1 and 11. Published by Kegan Paul, Trench, Trubner & Co., Ltd. 1926.

Celsus, Aulus Cornelius. Medicine: In Eight Books. Latin and English. Translated from L. Targa's Edition. Volume 1. London: E. Cox, St. Thomas's Street, Southwark. MDCCCXXX1.

Chadwick, John and Mann, W.N. *The Medical Works of Hippocrates.* A new translation from the original Greek. Blackwell's, Scientific Publications Oxford, 1950.

Chadwick, John and Mann, W.N. Edited by G.E.R. Lloyd. *Hippocratic Writings.* Penguin Books, 1978.

Cholmeley, Henry Patrick. John of Gaddesden and the Rosa Meducunae. Fiest Published in 1912, Reprint 2013 in India by Isha Books, New Delhi – 110009. ISBN 9789333164634.

Cooper, Samuel. *A New Dictionary of Practical Surgery containing a complete exhibition of the present state of Surgery, collected from the best and most original sources of information.* Dedicated to Dr Edward Roberts, FRS. Senior Physician to St. Bartholomew's Hospital. Printed for John Murray. 1809.

Cope, (Sir) Zachary. *The History of the Royal College of Surgeons of England.* Anthony Blond Ltd. 1959.

Cornford, F.M. *Before and After Socrates.* Published by the Syndics of the Cambridge University Press. Bentley house London, 1972.

Cornford, F.M. *From Religion to Philosophy: A study in the origins of Western speculation.* Dover Publications, Inc. New York. 2004. Originally Published, London by E. Arnold, 1912.

Crumplin, Michael FRCS. *Men of Steel. Surgery in the Napoleonic Wars.* Quiller Press, Shrewsbury, England. 207

Culpepper's Complete Herbal & English Physician. First Published by J. Gleave and Son, Deansgate, London 1826. Reproduced from the original by Harvey Sales 1981.

Dunster, Edward Swift. (1834–1888). *The History of Anaesthesia.* First published in 1875. Facsimile edition undated.

Ellis, Harold. *A History of Surgery.* Greenwich Medical media Ltd. 2001.

Ellis, Harold. *Operations that made History.* Cambridge University Press, Greenwich Medical Media, 1996.

Ellis, Harold. Calne, Sir Roy. Watson, Christopher. *General Surgery Lecture Notes.* Wiley-Blackwell. 2011.

Edwin Smith
Surgical Papyrus (Volume 1 of 2): Published in facsimle and hieroglyphic translation by James Edward Breasted. The University of Chicago Press, 1980.

Feinberg T.E. and Mallatt J.M. *The Ancient Origins of Consciousness. How the brain created experience.* The MIT Press, Cambridge, Massachusetts. 2017. ISBN. 9780262034333. P.40.

Freeman Charles. *The Greek Achievement. The Foundation of the Western World.* Allen lane. The penguin Press. 1999.

Gale, Thomas. 1507–1587. *Certaine VVorkes of Chirurgerie.* Hall, Rowlands, D. Printer 1563. Reprinted Boston Medical Library, in the Francis A. Countway Library of Medicine – Boston.

Galen of Pergamum. *On the Natural Faculties.* Theophania Publishing. Printed in USA. ISBN. 9781468024043.

Glubb, John Bagot (Glubb Pasha). *The Life and Times of Muhammad.* Hoddar and Stoughton. 1970.

Harding-Rains, A.J. & Richie, D. *Bailey & Love's Short Practice of Surgery.* Publisher H.K. Lewis & Co. Ltd. 1977. ISB. 0 7186 0431 8.

Harvey, William. *The Anatomical Exercises and De Motu Cordis (1627) & De Circulatione Sanguinis (1649)* in English Translation. Edited by Geoffrey Keynes. Dover Publications, Inc, New York 1995. ISBN. 13. 978-0-486-68827-5.

Harris C.R.S. *The Heart and Vascular System in Ancient Greek Medicine.* Oxford University Press. 1973. ISBN 0-19-858135-1.

Henry, John. *The Scientific Revolution and the origins of Modern Science.* First Published by Palgrave, ISBN 0-333-96090-4. 2002.

Herodotus. The Histories. Penguin Classics. Translated by Aubrey de Selincourt. Revised Edition 1972.

History of Medicine by Max Newburger. Translated by Ernest Playfair. Volume 1. Oxford University Press. 1910. Classic Reprint Series, 2015.

Hobsley, Michael. *Pathways in Surgical Management.* Edward Arnold Publishers, London 1979. ISBN 0-7131-4306-1.

Homer. The Iliad. Translated into English prose by Andrew Lang, Walter Leaf and Ernest Myers. Publisher: Macmillan and Co Ltd, London, 1912.

Homer. The Odyssey. Translated by C.V. Rieu. Guild Publishing London. 1946.
Hunter, John. *A Treatise on the Blood, Inflammation and Gun-Shot Wounds. Foreword by Everard Home.* Volume 1. Printed in Philadelphia in 1796. www.hansebooks.com

Hunter, John (Deceased). A Treatise on the Blood, Inflammation and Gun-shot Wounds. To which is Prefixed a Short account of the Authos's Life by his brother-in-law, Everard Home. Volume 2. Philadelphia: Published by Thomas Bradford, Printer. No. 8 South Front Street. 1796. Gale Ecco print Edition.

al-Khalili, Jim. Pathfinders. The Golden Age of Arabic Science. Published in Penguin Books 2012. ISBN 978-0-141-03836-0.

Kitto H.D.F. *The Greeks.* A Pelican Book. 1957.

Kolbert, Elizabeth. *The Sixth Extinction. An Unnatural History. Printed Picador ISBN 978-1-250-06218-5. 2014.*

Lee, Alex. Aur. Cor. Celsus. *On Medicine: In Eight Books,* Latin and English. A.M., Surg. 1831

Lindberg, David C. *The Beginnings of Western Science. The European Scientific Tradition in Philosophical, Religious and Institutional Context, 600 BC to AD 1450.* The University of Chicago Press, 1992.

Lloyd. G.E.R. *Ancient Culture and Society. Early Greek Science: Thales to Aristotle.* Chatto and Windus, London 1982.

Lloyd G.E.R. *Greek science after Aristotle.* W.W. Norton and Company, London, 1973.

Lloyd, G.E.R. Aristotle: *The Growth and Structure of his Thought.* Cambridge University press. 1968.

Majno, G. *The Healing Hand: Man and Wound in the Ancient World.* Harvard University Press 1975.

Maybury, Nigel Keith. *The End of the Golden Age of General Surgery. 1870–2000. The Training and Practice of a general Surgeon in the late Twentieth Century.* ISBN 1499531370 and ISBN 13: 9781499531374. 2014. Amazon.

Moore, Wendy. The Knife Man: Blood, Body-Snatching and the Birth of Modern Surgery. Bantam Books 2005.

Newburger, Max. History of Medicine. Volume 1 of 2, Part 1. Translated by Ernest Playfair. London. Oxford University Press. 1910. Forgotten Books Republished 2015.

Overy, Richard, Editor. The Times History of the World. Published in 1999 for Times Books. ISBN 0-00-761900-6.

Paget, Stephen. Paget, Sir James and Hart, Ernest. Masters of Medicine. John Hunter, Man of Science and Surgeon (1728–1793). Leopold Classic Library. Reprint. First Printed in MDCCCXCV11.

Parker, G. The Early History of Surgery in Great Britain. Its Organisation and Development. 1920. A & C Black, Soho Square, London.

Parkinson, James. Hunterian Reminiscences, Being the Substance of a Course of Lectures on the Principles and Practice of Surgery Delivered by John Hunter in the Year 1785. Taken in shorthand by Mr James Parkinson and published by Sherwood, Gilbert, and Piper, Paternoster Row, London 1893. Nabu Public Domain Reprints.

Pepys, Samuel. The Diary of Samuel Pepys. Editor Robert Latham. Penguin Classics. 2003.

Perutz, Max. Is Science Necessary. Essays on science and scientists. E.P. Dutton, New York. 1989

Petechuk, David. Organ Transplantation. Health and medical issues today. Greenwood press, Westport, Connecticut. 2006.

Pormann, Peter E. The Oriental Tradition of Paul of Aegina's Pragmateia. Brill, Leiden and Boston, 2004.

Pormann, Peter E. & Savage-Smith, Emily. Medieval Islamic Medicine. Edinburgh University Press. 2010. ISBN 978 0 7486 2067 8.

Porter, Roy, Editor. The Cambridge Illustrated History of Medicine. Cambridge University Press 1996.

Power, D'Arcy. William Harvey 1578–1657. Printed by Amazon.

Principe, Lawrence M. The Scientific Revolution. A very short introduction. 2011. OUP.

Rice, Dr Tony. Voyages of Discovery. Three Centuries of Natural History Exploration. 2000. The Natural History Museum, London. ISBN 1-902686-02-0.

Russel Bertrand. History of Western Philosophy George Allen and Unwin Ltd. London. 1947.

Sarton, George. Galen of Pergamon. Third Series of Logan Clendening Lectures on the History and Philosophy of Medicine. University of Kansas Press 1954.

Shapin, Steven. The Scientific Revolution. The University of Chicago Press. 1996.

Sigerist, Henry E. A History of Medicine. Volume 11. Early Greek, Hindu and Persian Medicine. Oxford University Press. 1961. ISBN: 978-0-19-505079-0.

Singer, Charles. Galen on Anatomical Procedures. Translation of surviving books with introduction and notes. Oxford University Press. 1956. ISBN. 0-19-924116-7.

Spencer, W.G. CELSUS on Medicine. Books 1–4, 5–6 and Books 7–8. Loeb Classical Library. Harvard University Press 1935.

Soranus' Gynaecology, Translated by Owsei Temkin. The Johns Hopkins University Press, Baltimore, USA. Paperback Edition, 1991.

Tait, Lawson. Lectures on Ectopic Pregnancy and Pelvic Haematocele. Leopold Classic Library. Facsimile First Printed in 1888.

Taylor, A.E. ARISTOTLE. Dover Publications Inc., N.Y. 1955.

The Times. History of the World. New Edition. Edited by Geoffrey Barraclough and new Edition edited by Richard Overy. First Published in 1999 by Times Books. Harper Collins Publishers.

Thompson, D'Arcy Wentworth. On Growth and Form. First Published in 1917. Republished Stellar Editions 2016.

Thorwold, Jurgen. Science and Secrets of Early Medicine. Egypt, Mesopotamia, India, China, Mexico, Peru. Thames and Hudson London, 1962.

Treves, Sir Frederick and Jonathan Hutchinson. A Manual of Operative Surgery. Volumes 1 and 2. Forgotten Books. Com. ISBN 978-1-330-29953-1. Originally published by Lea and Febiger, Philadelphia and New York 1910.

Underwood. E. Ashworth, Editor of Essays in Honour of Charles Singer. Science Medicine and History. Essays on the Evolution of Scientific Thought and Medical practice. Volumes One and Two. Oxford University Press 1953.

Wiseman Richard. Several Chirurgical Treatises. 1686. Early History of Medicine, Health and Disease. Printed by R. Norton and J. Maycock. Microfilmed 1979.

Wiseman, Richard. Surgeon and Sergeant-Surgeon to Charles II. A Biographical Study (1891) by Thomas Longmore. Publishers Longmans, Green, and Co. Kessinger Legacy Reprints. 2018
www.Kessinger.Net

Ziccardi, M. James. Medieval Philosophy: A Practical Guide to Roger Bacon. Copyright M. James Zicardi, 2011. ISBN: 13: 978-1466418325.

Index